Serenity & Strength: Stretching Exercises for Seniors

Rediscover Life's Vitality Over 60: Simple Guide to Combat Stiffness, Improve Flexibility, Boost Mobility and Avoid Injury with 20 Minutes a Day!

By

Evelyn Grace

Table of Contents

Introduction

Welcome, dear reader, to a journey of rejuvenation! A journey that doesn't count the candles on your birthday cake but values the vigor in your spirit. Here, you've embarked on an adventure—a defiance against age-old stereotypes, a proclamation that the golden years can indeed be golden.

Life is a rich tapestry, each thread a unique story, a distinct rhythm. The dance of life may slow as the years roll on, but it never truly stops. This book? It's your dance partner, guiding you step by step, ensuring your dance is filled with grace and vitality. Our bodies are marvels of intricate machinery, designed for movement, expression, experiencing the world in all its multifaceted glory. As the years stack up, the machinery seeks tender care, a gentle stretch, a nudge to keep the wheels turning, the music playing.

Simplicity and adaptability are the essences of this book. Tailored for seniors from all walks of life, whether you are a seasoned fitness enthusiast or a curious beginner, the ensuing pages offer knowledge, warmth, and a dash of humor, making the journey enjoyable and sustainable.

Why stretching, you might wonder? The answer is woven into every muscle, every joint, every fiber of our being. Stretching is the harmonizing melody between body and mind, a gentle whisper awakening dormant potentials, a bridge to realms of vitality and tranquility.

The chapters ahead delve deep into the science and art of stretching, shedding light on its myriad benefits for seniors. From enhancing flexibility to fostering mental well-being, from alleviating aches to nurturing balance—the spectrum of benefits is as diverse as it is profound.

Safety is our guiding compass. Each exercise, each piece of advice, each wisdom nugget is framed within the bounds of caution and body awareness. Your journey is unique; thus, tuning into your body, adapting routines, and savoring the process become the golden threads weaving this tapestry. As we traverse the realms of stretching, we encounter real stories, anecdotes of triumphs and challenges, reflections on human resilience and adaptability. These narratives are the heartbeat of the book, resonating with the universal rhythm of life's dance.

In the world of stretching, every movement and moment of rest is crucial. Just like a well-curated playlist can set the tone for your day, the varied exercises in this book are tailored for different needs and goals. Whether you're aiming for a simple stretch to start the day or a full-body workout, this guide offers practical, step-by-step routines to help you feel your best, both physically and mentally. This isn't just a guide; it's a companion, a friend accompanying you through the valleys and peaks of senior stretching. It's a celebration of the human spirit, a testament to the timeless beauty of movement, a melody of hope and strength.

So, let's dance through the pages, push boundaries, and weave a tapestry of vitality, grace, and joy. Welcome to a stretching journey, a rediscovery, a celebration of life's golden rhythm.

Chapter 1: Foundations of Stretching for Seniors

Embarking on a journey into the world of stretching, especially designed for seniors, is like opening a door to a realm of vitality, grace, and well-being. This chapter lays the cornerstone, unveiling the essential elements and principles of stretching, meticulously tailored to meet the unique needs and aspirations of seniors. Here, we unravel the tapestry of knowledge, fostering a deeper understanding and appreciation of the transformative power of stretching.

1.1 Importance of Stretching for Seniors

Golden years? More like the 'Stretchy Platinum Era'! Remember those early morning stretches we used to do just to get the cricks out? Now, in our prime years, every stretch is like a mini-adventure, a small victory, a tiny dance party. Think of it as your body's way of saying, "Hey, I've still got the moves!"

Stretching isn't just about reaching for your toes; it's about reaching out to life. For us seniors, it's like having a secret weapon against the sneaky stiffness that tries to set in. Every time you stretch, it's as if you're telling those joints, "Not today!" It's about bending so you don't break, swaying in the rhythm of life, and maybe, just maybe, showing off to the grandkids.

But wait, there's more! Stretching is like that trusty old radio - it tunes out the static (read: aches and pains) and tunes into the golden hits. And by hits, we mean those feel-good endorphins. It's a daily dose of 'feel-awesome' without any side effects, unless you count increased flexibility and a pep in your step as side effects.

And here's the kicker: stretching is also a mind game. It's a mental high-five, a pat on the back, and a gentle reminder that, "Hey, you've still got it!" It bridges the gap between mind and body, ensuring they're always on the same page, even if sometimes it feels like they're reading different books.

In this chapter, we'll peel back the layers of stretching, but not in a boring, textbook way. We'll journey through its twists, turns, and "Aha!" moments. We'll dive into why it feels so darn good and how it stealthily sneaks benefits into our lives.

Stretching is more than just an activity; it's a lifestyle, a celebration, a daily toast to our enduring spirit. So, here's to making every stretch count, to laughing in the face of stiffness, and to always, always dancing like everyone (or no one) is watching.

To wrap it up, stretching in our golden years is like adding sprinkles to a sundae. Not necessary, but oh, it makes life so much more colorful! Dive into this chapter, and let's journey together through the fun, frolic, and flexibility of stretching. Cheers to our 'Stretchy Platinum Era'!

1.2 Benefits of Regular Stretching

Embarking on a regular stretching routine unfolds a plethora of benefits, particularly for seniors whose bodies and lifestyles have transitioned over the years. The advantages are immediate and long-term, impacting physical well-being, mental health, and overall quality of life.

Enhanced Flexibility and Range of Motion: The first and most discernible benefit is improved flexibility. Regular stretching lengthens the muscles and increases the range of motion in the joints, making daily activities like reaching, bending, and turning smoother and more effortless.

Reduced Muscle Stiffness and Tension: Age often brings stiffness and tension. Stretching alleviates these conditions, promoting relaxation and easing discomfort, allowing seniors to enjoy a more active and pain-free lifestyle.

Increased Blood Circulation: Stretching boosts blood flow to the muscles. This enhanced circulation brings more nutrients to the muscles and removes waste byproducts, fostering healthier and more efficient muscle function.

Improved Posture and Balance: Regular stretching strengthens muscles and enhances body awareness. This dual benefit helps in maintaining an upright posture and improving balance, essential factors in preventing falls and related injuries in seniors.

Stress Relief and Mental Calmness: The act of stretching is not just physical. It's a moment of mindfulness, a time of inward focus that calms the mind, reduces stress, and contributes to mental well-being.

Enhanced Coordination: Synchronized muscle actions are crucial for movement efficiency. Regular stretching fosters better coordination, ensuring that different body parts work harmoniously.

Injury Prevention: By increasing flexibility and reducing muscle tension, stretching indirectly helps in preventing injuries. It prepares the body for physical activity, making muscles less prone to strain and tears.

Supports Healthy Joint Function: Stretching maintains the range of motion in the joints and reduces stiffness, essential for healthy joint function and mobility.

Promotion of Overall Health: Beyond the muscles and joints, stretching has a holistic impact. It contributes to better sleep, boosts immune function, and enhances overall well-being.

Community and Social Interaction: Joining stretching classes or groups fosters a sense of community. It's an opportunity for social interaction, sharing experiences, and building connections, combating feelings of isolation.

Incorporating regular stretching into daily routines is not a monumental task. It's about small, consistent steps. A stretch here, a bend there, gradually woven into the fabric of everyday life. It's about making it a habit, a part of the morning routine, or a way to unwind in the evening.

For seniors, the journey of stretching is also about rediscovery. It's about reconnecting with the body, understanding its rhythm, and respecting its limits. It's about finding joy in movement, celebrating small victories, and embracing the progress made each day.

Practicality is key. The stretching routine doesn't have to be elaborate or time-consuming. It's about finding what works, what feels good, and what brings benefits. It's about listening to the body, adapting the stretches to individual needs, and enjoying the journey.

The benefits of regular stretching are manifold and significant. They touch upon various aspects of life, improving physical health, enhancing mental well-being, and fostering social connections. For seniors seeking a balanced and fulfilling life, incorporating stretching into their routine is a step worth taking. The rewards are tangible, the effort is modest, and the journey is enriching.

1.3 Safety Guidelines

Embarking on a stretching routine, especially for seniors, necessitates a thoughtful approach to safety. This subchapter, "Safety Guidelines," sheds light on practical, straightforward, and crucial tips to ensure that your stretching journey is not only fruitful but also safe and enjoyable.

Start Slowly and Gently: Remember, it's not a race. Begin with gentle stretches and gradually intensify the routine. Listen to your body, understand its pace, and don't rush the process.

Warm-Up is Essential: Before diving into stretching, warm up your body. A brisk walk or marching in place for a few minutes can do the trick. It prepares your muscles and joints, making them more pliable and less prone to injury.

Pain is a Red Flag: A golden rule – stretching should never cause pain. If it does, it's a signal to stop immediately. Feel the stretch, but if it crosses over to pain, you've gone too far. Respect your body's boundaries.

Breathe Freely and Deeply: Your breath is your guide. Never hold your breath during stretches. Inhale deeply, exhale slowly. It keeps the oxygen flowing, which is essential for muscle function.

Maintain Proper Form: It's not about how far you can stretch, but how well you can hold the stretch. Keep your spine aligned, don't lock your joints, and avoid bouncing. Quality over quantity, always.

Consistency Over Intensity: Regular, consistent stretching is far more effective and safer than intense, infrequent sessions. It's about building a habit, not pushing the limits in one go.

Hydrate and Nourish: Your body needs fuel. Stay hydrated, eat balanced meals, and ensure you're well-nourished. It aids muscle recovery and overall well-being.

Use Support if Needed: Don't hesitate to use props like chairs, belts, or walls for support. It aids balance and stability, especially important for seniors.

Know Your Health Status: Be aware of your medical conditions, medications, and overall health status. Consult your healthcare provider before starting a new stretching routine, especially if you have existing health issues.

Celebrate Small Victories: Every stretch, every session is a step forward. Celebrate the progress, no matter how small. It builds motivation and a positive mindset.

Safety is paramount. It's the foundation upon which your stretching journey is built. By following these guidelines, not only do you protect your body, but you also ensure that each stretch, each session, brings you closer to your goals in a healthy, enjoyable manner. Remember, it's your journey, your body. Respect it, enjoy the process, and the benefits will surely follow.

Chapter 2: Upper Body Stretches

2.1 Neck and Shoulder Stretches

NECK TILTS

Description & Benefit: The Neck Tilts exercise is a simple yet effective movement designed to stretch the side muscles of the neck, known as the sternocleidomastoid and scalene muscles. Regular practice can increase neck flexibility, reduce tension, and alleviate discomfort caused by stiffness or prolonged static postures, such as sitting at a desk.

Instructions:

1. Starting Position: Sit up straight in a comfortable chair with your feet flat on the floor. Place your hands on your lap and relax your shoulders (or use your hands to execute the exercise as shown in the picture below).
2. Movement: Slowly tilt your head to one side, bringing your ear closer to your shoulder. Keep your eyes facing forward.
3. Duration: Hold the tilt for 15-30 seconds, feeling a gentle stretch along the side of the neck.
4. Return: Slowly lift your head back to the center and upright position.
5. Repetition: Repeat the tilt on the opposite side. Perform 2-3 sets on each side.

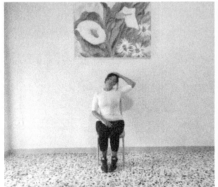 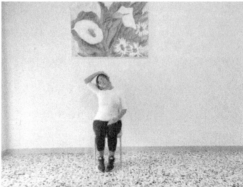

Tips:

- Ensure you're not raising your shoulder to meet your ear; the movement should come solely from your neck.
- Keep the rest of your body still and avoid any sudden jerky movements to prevent strain.

12

- Breathe deeply and regularly throughout the exercise. Avoid holding your breath.

Alternative exercises:

- Neck Rotations: From a neutral position, gently turn your head to one side, bringing your chin towards your shoulder. Hold, then return to center and repeat on the other side.
- Chin Tucks: Sitting upright, gently tuck your chin to your chest, feeling a stretch along the back of your neck.

SCAN the QR for the Video Bonus

SHOULDER ROLLS

Description & Benefit: Shoulder Rolls are a foundational exercise to enhance mobility in the shoulder girdle. They help in releasing tension and tightness accumulated from daily activities or prolonged postures. Regularly incorporating shoulder rolls can lead to reduced stiffness, improved posture, and increased circulation to the upper body.

Instructions:

1. Starting Position: Sit comfortably in an upright position, either on a chair or on the floor. Keep your spine elongated, feet flat on the ground (if seated on a chair).
2. Movement: Begin by lifting both shoulders up towards your ears in a shrugging motion.
3. Continuation: From the elevated position, roll your shoulders back, squeezing the shoulder blades together.
4. Completion: Continue the rolling motion by bringing the shoulders down and then forward to the starting position.
5. Duration: Complete this circular roll for about 10-15 repetitions.

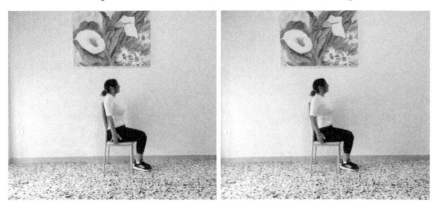

Tips:

- Keep the movement smooth and controlled; avoid any abrupt or jerky actions.
- Focus on the full range of motion, ensuring you're hitting the up, back, down, and forward positions distinctly.
- Use your breath to enhance the stretch. Inhale as you lift the shoulders, and exhale as you complete the roll.

14

Alternative exercises:

- Shoulder Shrug: Simply lift both shoulders towards your ears and hold for a few seconds before releasing. It's a great way to release tension quickly.

- Scapular Squeeze: With arms at your sides, squeeze your shoulder blades together as if you're trying to hold a pencil between them. This helps in strengthening the muscles between the shoulder blades.

SCAN the QR for the Video Bonus

NECK ROTATION

Description & Benefit: Neck Rotations target the cervical spine, providing relief from tension and increasing the range of motion. By performing this exercise regularly, one can reduce the risk of neck pain, strain, and even headaches. It's an essential exercise for those who spend long hours working at desks, on computers, or driving.

Instructions:

1. Starting Position: Sit or stand with a straight spine, ensuring your head is aligned with your spine and not jutting forward.
2. Movement: Slowly turn your head to the right, aiming to look over your right shoulder. Only go as far as is comfortable.
3. Hold: Once you've reached your comfortable limit, hold the position for 5-10 seconds, feeling a gentle stretch on the left side of your neck.
4. Return: Slowly bring your head back to the center position.
5. Repeat: Now, turn your head to the left, aiming to look over your left shoulder. Hold for 5-10 seconds.
6. Duration: Perform this rotation 5 times on each side.

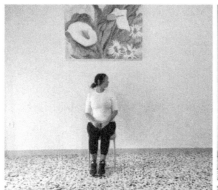 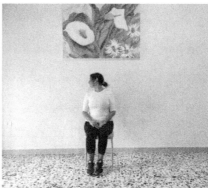

Tips:

- Ensure the movement is slow and controlled. Avoid any quick or forceful rotations.
- Keep your shoulders relaxed and down. They shouldn't rise or tense up during the rotations.
- If you feel any sharp pain, stop immediately and consult a healthcare professional.

Alternative exercises:

- Chin Tucks: Sitting or standing tall, tuck your chin into your chest without bending your spine. This exercise stretches the back of your neck.
- Neck Flexion and Extension: Start by looking straight ahead. Slowly tilt your head back to look up to the ceiling (extension) and then down towards your chest (flexion).
- Lateral Neck Stretch: Keeping your head upright, tilt it to one side as if trying to touch your ear to your shoulder. This targets the side muscles of the neck.

SCAN the QR for the Video Bonus

SHOULDER SHRUG STRETCH

Description & Benefit: The Shoulder Shrug Stretch primarily targets the trapezius muscles located at the top of your shoulders. This exercise aids in releasing tension built up from daily activities like typing, driving, or carrying bags. By routinely performing this stretch, you can alleviate shoulder and upper back stiffness, enhancing overall mobility.

Instructions:

1. Starting Position: Stand or sit with a straight spine, feet shoulder-width apart if standing.
2. Movement: Elevate both your shoulders towards your ears, as if you're shrugging.
3. Hold: Keep your shoulders lifted, squeezing them as you maintain this "shrugged" position for 5-10 seconds.
4. Release: Slowly lower your shoulders back down, feeling a stretch in the upper trapezius muscles.
5. Duration: Repeat this process for a total of 5-7 times.

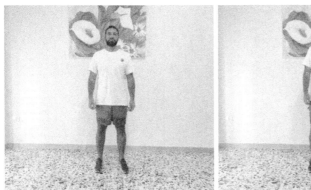 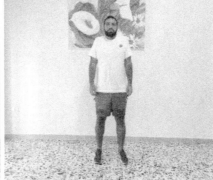

Tips:

- Ensure that your movements are controlled and deliberate, avoiding any jerky motions.
- As you elevate your shoulders, avoid pushing your head forward. Keep it neutral.
- Remember to breathe. Inhale as you lift your shoulders and exhale as you release them.

Alternative exercises:

- Shoulder Rolls: While either sitting or standing, roll your shoulders forward in a circular motion, then reverse the direction, rolling them backward.
- Neck Tilts: From a neutral position, tilt your head to one side, trying to bring your ear to your shoulder. This will stretch the opposing side's trapezius muscle.

- Scapular Squeeze: With your arms at your sides, squeeze your shoulder blades together as if holding a pencil between them. This targets the rhomboids and middle trapezius muscles.

SCAN the QR for the Video Bonus

2.2 Arm and Wrist Stretches

WRIST FLEXOR STRETCH

Description & Benefit: The Wrist Flexor Stretch is primarily aimed at lengthening the flexor muscles located on the underside of the forearm. These muscles are often under strain from activities such as typing, writing, or even carrying objects. By stretching them regularly, you can reduce the risk of wrist strain, carpal tunnel syndrome, and maintain a healthy range of motion in the wrist joint.

Instructions:

1. Starting Position: Extend your arm in front of you with your palm facing up.
2. Movement: With your other hand, gently press on the fingers of the extended hand, directing them towards the floor.
3. Hold: Maintain this position, ensuring a gentle pull is felt on the underside of the forearm. Hold for 15-30 seconds.
4. Release: Slowly release the pressure and relax the wrist.
5. Duration: Repeat the process 2-3 times for each wrist.

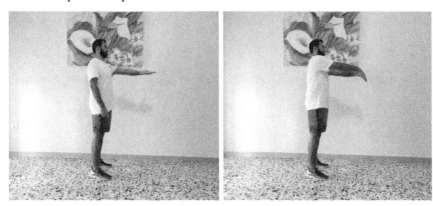

Tips:

- Make sure you're stretching gently, especially if you're new to the exercise. Overstretching can cause discomfort or injury.
- If you feel any sharp pain, immediately stop the stretch.
- Ensure a straight alignment of the arm during the stretch for maximum benefit.

Alternative exercises:

- Wrist Extensor Stretch: Similar to the flexor stretch, but with the palm facing down. Press on the back of the hand, pushing the fingers towards the floor.

- Wrist Rotation: Extend your arm and rotate your wrist in a circular motion, both clockwise and counter-clockwise.

- Prayer Stretch: Join your palms together in front of your chest, like a prayer position. Lower the palms towards the waist while keeping the hands close to the chest, feeling a stretch in the wrists.

SCAN the QR for the Video Bonus

TRICEP STRETCH

Description & Benefit: The Tricep Stretch primarily targets the tricep muscles located at the back of the upper arm. These muscles are crucial for actions that involve pushing or throwing. Regularly stretching the triceps can help improve arm mobility, reduce tightness, and prevent injuries, especially for those who engage in activities that heavily involve arm movements.

Instructions:

1. Starting Position: Stand or sit upright.
2. Movement: Raise one arm overhead, and then bend the elbow, bringing the hand down towards the opposite shoulder blade.
3. Support: With the opposite hand, gently press on the bent elbow, enhancing the stretch.
4. Hold: Maintain this position, ensuring a gentle pull is felt along the back of your upper arm. Hold for 15-30 seconds.
5. Release: Slowly release the elbow and return the arm to its resting position.
6. Duration: Repeat the process 2-3 times for each arm.

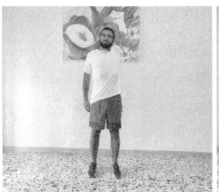 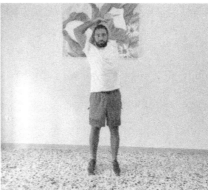

Tips:

- Ensure you keep your spine straight during the stretch.

- Stretch to the point of tension, not pain. If you feel any sharp pain, stop immediately.

- Breathe deeply and evenly throughout the stretch.

Alternative exercises:

- Bicep Stretch: Extend your arms behind you, interlocking your fingers. Slowly lift your arms up until you feel a stretch in your biceps and chest.

- Forearm Stretch: Extend an arm out in front of you with the palm facing up. Using the opposite hand, gently press down on the extended hand's fingers, stretching the forearm.

- Shoulder Stretch: Extend one arm straight in front of you, then cross it over the chest. Using the opposite hand, gently pull the arm closer to the chest.

SCAN the QR for the Video Bonus

WRIST EXTENSOR STRETCH

Description & Benefit: The Wrist Extensor Stretch primarily focuses on the extensor muscles located on the top of the forearm. These muscles play a pivotal role in extending the wrist and fingers. Regularly stretching the wrist extensors can alleviate tightness, prevent overuse injuries, and maintain wrist flexibility, especially crucial for those who frequently use their hands, such as typists or musicians.

Instructions:

1. Starting Position: Sit or stand with your spine in a neutral position.
2. Movement: Extend one arm straight out in front of you with your palm facing down.
3. Stretch: Using the opposite hand, gently press down on the outstretched hand until you feel a stretch along the top of your forearm.
4. Hold: Maintain this position, feeling a gentle but consistent stretch. Hold for 15-30 seconds.
5. Release: Gently release the pressure and let the wrist return to its natural position.
6. Duration: Repeat the stretch 2-3 times for each wrist.

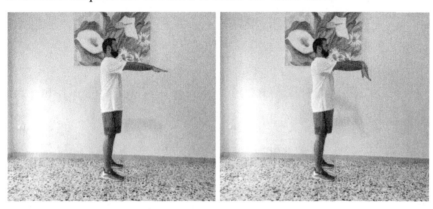

Tips:

- Ensure you keep your shoulder relaxed during the stretch.
- Always stretch to the point of mild tension, not pain. If you encounter any sharp or acute pain, cease the stretch immediately.
- Engage in deep, consistent breathing throughout the stretch to facilitate relaxation and effectiveness.

22

Alternative exercises:

- Wrist Flexor Stretch: Extend your arm out with the palm facing up. Using your opposite hand, gently press the fingers of the outstretched hand towards the floor, stretching the muscles on the underside of the forearm.

- Finger Tendon Glide: Start with fingers extended straight out. Then make a hook fist; return to a straight hand. Make a full fist; return to a straight hand. Make a straight fist; return to a straight hand.

- Prayer Stretch: Place your palms together in front of your chest, fingers pointing upwards. Lower the hands while keeping the heels of the hands touching, feeling a stretch in the wrists.

SCAN the QR for the Video Bonus

2.3 Back Stretches

CAT-COW STRETCH

Description & Benefit: The Cat-Cow Stretch is a yoga-derived movement that targets the spine, specifically the thoracic and lumbar regions. It promotes flexibility, can help improve posture, and aids in spinal fluid circulation, ensuring that nutrients reach the discs between the vertebrae. The alternating arching and rounding of the back also provide a gentle massage to the organs in the abdomen, aiding in digestion and stimulating the kidneys.

Instructions:

1. Starting Position: Begin on your hands and knees in a tabletop position. Ensure your wrists are directly under your shoulders and your knees are directly under your hips. Your back should be flat and your gaze towards the floor.

2. Cat Pose: Exhale deeply. Round your spine towards the ceiling, tucking your chin to your chest and drawing your belly button towards your spine. Feel the stretch along the back.

3. Cow Pose: As you inhale, arch your back, lifting your head and tailbone towards the ceiling. Allow your belly to sink towards the floor, and feel the stretch along the front of your torso.

4. Flow: Continue flowing between the Cat and Cow poses for 8-10 cycles, synchronizing the movement with your breath.

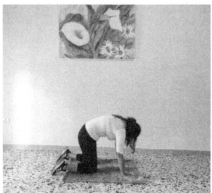 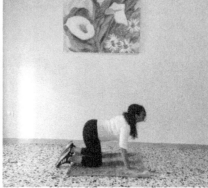

Tips:

- Engage your abdominal muscles throughout the exercise to support the spine.
- Ensure your movements are smooth and controlled, flowing seamlessly from one pose to the other.

- Keep your hands flat on the ground, spreading your fingers to distribute your weight evenly across the palms.
- If you have wrist discomfort, consider using yoga blocks under your hands or doing the exercise on your fists.

Alternative exercises:

- Child's Pose: From a kneeling position, sit back on your heels, stretch your arms out in front, and lower your forehead to the ground.
- Puppy Pose: Starting on all fours, keep your hips over your knees and walk your hands forward, lowering your chest towards the ground.
- Spinal Twist: Lying on your back, bring one knee into your chest and then guide it across your body with the opposite hand, keeping both shoulders flat on the floor.

SEATED TWIST STRETCH

Description & Benefit: The Seated Twist Stretch, often recognized from yoga practices, is a powerful movement that primarily targets the muscles of the spine, obliques, and shoulders. It aids in improving spinal flexibility, promoting digestion, and can alleviate stiffness in the back. Twisting motions also support detoxification in the body by massaging internal organs, leading to better circulation and removal of waste products.

Instructions:

1. Starting Position: Begin by sitting on the floor with your legs extended straight in front of you.
2. Initiate the Twist: Bend your right knee, placing your right foot outside of your left thigh. Ensure your right buttock remains on the floor.
3. Deepen the Stretch: Place your right hand on the floor behind you for support. Inhale and lift your left arm towards the sky. As you exhale, twist to your right, placing your left elbow on the outside of your right knee. Turn your head to look over your right shoulder.
4. Hold & Release: Maintain this position, ensuring you sit tall with each inhale and twist a little deeper with each exhale. Hold for 20-30 seconds, then slowly unwind and repeat on the opposite side.

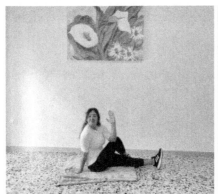 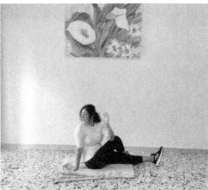

Tips:

- Always engage your core muscles during the twist to protect your spine.
- Ensure you're twisting from the base of your spine upwards, not just turning your neck.
- For a deeper stretch, try drawing your bent knee closer to your chest.
- Remember to breathe deeply and evenly throughout the stretch.

Alternative exercises:

- Supine Twist: Lying on your back, draw both knees into your chest. Keep your shoulders flat on the ground as you drop your knees to one side, turning your head to the opposite side.
- Standing Twist: Stand tall, feet hip-width apart. Twist your torso to one side, allowing your arms to swing naturally, and then twist to the other side.
- Chair Twist: Sit sideways on a chair, holding onto the backrest. Keep your feet flat on the ground and twist your torso, pulling against the backrest to deepen the stretch.

CHILD'S POSE STRETCH

Description & Benefit: Child's Pose, known as "Balasana" in Sanskrit, is a foundational yoga pose that serves as a resting posture. It primarily stretches the back, hips, thighs, and ankles while relaxing the spine, shoulders, and neck. This pose is not just a physical stretch but also a mental reprieve, offering a moment of introspection, relaxation, and relief from daily stresses. The posture promotes circulation to the muscles of the spine and can alleviate back and neck pain when done correctly.

Instructions:

1. Starting Position: Begin on your hands and knees in a tabletop position. Ensure your wrists are directly below your shoulders and your knees below your hips.
2. Initiate the Stretch: Exhale and lower your hips back towards your heels. Extend your arms out in front of you.
3. Deepen the Stretch: Let your forehead gently rest on the floor. If needed, you can place a cushion or folded blanket under your forehead for comfort.
4. Hold & Release: Remain in this position for 1-3 minutes, breathing deeply. To exit the pose, gently lift your forehead and walk your hands back towards your knees, returning to a seated position.

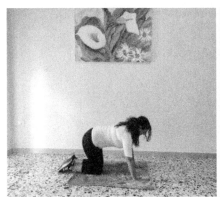 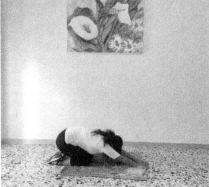

Tips:

- Keep your arms extended and active, reaching out to fully stretch the back.
- If your buttocks don't reach your heels, place a cushion or folded blanket between them for support.
- Breathe deeply, directing your breath into the back of your ribcage to enhance the stretch and relaxation.
- For those with knee concerns, consider placing a folded blanket under the knees for added cushioning.

Alternative exercises:

- Extended Puppy Pose: From a tabletop position, keep your hips over your knees and walk your hands forward, lowering your chest towards the ground.

- Sphinx Pose: Lie on your stomach, prop yourself up on your forearms, ensuring your elbows are under your shoulders. Press down through the palms and lift your chest up, stretching the spine.

- Thread the Needle: Starting in a tabletop position, slide your right arm under your left with the palm facing up. Allow your right shoulder and temple to rest on the ground, stretching the upper back and shoulder.

SCAN the QR for the Video Bonus

Chapter 3: Lower Body Stretches

3.1 Stretching the Hips and Glutes

GENTLE PIGEON POSE

Description & Benefit: The Gentle Pigeon Pose is a modified version of the traditional pigeon pose in yoga. It focuses on stretching the hip rotators and flexors, providing relief from tightness in the lower back and hips. Regularly practicing this pose can improve hip flexibility, reduce pain, and enhance overall lower body mobility, making it especially beneficial for seniors.

Instructions:

1. Begin by sitting on a mat with your legs stretched out in front of you.
2. Bend your right leg, bringing the heel towards the left hip, laying your right shin on the mat.
3. Extend your left leg straight back, toes pointing.
4. Keep your hips square to the front and distribute weight evenly.
5. Place your hands on either side of your hips, fingers facing forward.
6. Sit up tall, elongating the spine. Deepen the stretch by gently leaning forward from the hips, keeping the spine straight.
7. Hold for 20-30 seconds, breathing deeply.
8. Slowly return to the starting position and switch legs.

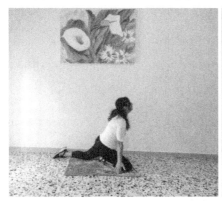 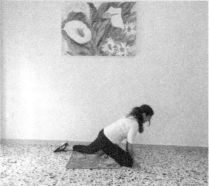

Tips:

- Use a folded blanket or cushion under your right hip (the one in front) if you find it hovering above the ground. This provides support and ensures proper alignment.

- Avoid leaning to one side; keep weight distributed evenly.
- If you have knee issues, be extra cautious and ensure there's no pain in the bent knee.

Alternative exercises:

- Seated Hip Stretch: Sitting on a chair, cross your right ankle over your left knee and gently press down on the right knee while leaning forward.
- Butterfly Stretch: Sit on the ground, bring the soles of your feet together, and gently press your knees towards the ground.
- Hip Circles: Stand with feet hip-width apart and hands on hips, then move your hips in circular motions.
- Lying Hip Stretch: Lie on your back, bend your knees, and cross your right ankle over your left knee, gently pulling the left knee towards your chest.

CHAIR-BASED HIP OPENER

Description & Benefit: The Chair-Based Hip Opener is a gentle yet effective exercise tailored for seniors or individuals with limited mobility. By utilizing a chair for support, this exercise helps stretch the hip flexors and inner thighs, promoting better hip and lower back flexibility. Regularly practicing this pose can alleviate hip tightness, improve range of motion, and counteract the effects of prolonged sitting.

Instructions:

1. Begin by sitting at the front edge of a sturdy chair, feet flat on the ground, hip-width apart.
2. Maintain an upright posture, with your spine straight and shoulders relaxed.
3. Carefully lift your right ankle and place it on your left thigh, just above the knee, allowing the right knee to drop open to the side.
4. Keep both sit bones anchored to the chair and press your right knee gently downwards.
5. For a deeper stretch, you can hinge at the hips and lean slightly forward, keeping the spine straight.
6. Hold for 20-30 seconds, taking deep breaths.
7. Slowly return to the starting position and switch to the other leg.

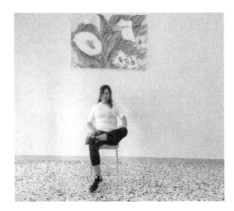

Tips:

- Ensure the chair is on a non-slip surface to prevent any movement.
- If your knee feels stressed or uncomfortable, place a cushion or folded towel under the lifted ankle.
- Always engage your core muscles slightly to maintain balance and protect your lower back.
- It's essential to keep the foot of the elevated leg flexed to protect the knee.

Alternative exercises:

- Seated Leg Cradle: While sitting on a chair, lift your right foot off the ground, cradle it with both hands under the knee and ankle, and gently pull it towards your chest.
- Ankle-on-Knee Pose: Sitting on the floor, bend both knees, place the right ankle over the left knee, and gently press the right knee towards the floor.
- Standing Hip Flexor Stretch: Stand behind a chair, hold onto the backrest, lift the right foot towards the glutes, and hold the ankle with the right hand.
- Seated Butterfly Stretch: Sit on the ground, bring the soles of your feet together, and gently press your knees towards the ground. Top of FormBottom of Form

UPLIFTING BRIDGES

Description & Benefit: Uplifting Bridges, commonly known as the bridge pose, is an essential exercise to strengthen the lower back, glutes, and hamstrings. It helps in enhancing core stability and improving posture. Seniors benefit from this exercise as it aids in alleviating lower back pain, enhancing hip mobility, and building a stronger core. Moreover, it helps in improving blood circulation and can be therapeutic for high blood pressure.

Instructions:

1. Start by lying flat on your back with knees bent and feet hip-width apart, placed firmly on the ground. Your arms should be resting by your sides, palms facing down.
2. Inhale deeply. While exhaling, press through your heels and gently lift your hips off the floor.
3. Engage your glutes, thighs, and core muscles as you elevate your pelvis towards the ceiling. Your body from the shoulder to the knees should form a straight line.
4. Hold the bridge position for 10-15 seconds while taking deep and controlled breaths.
5. Slowly lower your hips back to the starting position while inhaling.
6. Repeat the exercise 5-10 times, depending on your comfort level.

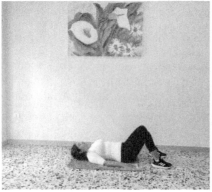 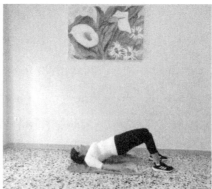

Tips:

- Ensure your feet are firmly planted, and your weight is evenly distributed between both feet.
- Avoid pressing your neck into the ground; instead, keep it relaxed.
- If you feel any strain in your neck or back, lower your hips and rest before attempting again.
- Always engage your core muscles to maintain stability and protect your lower back.

Alternative exercises:

- Single-leg Bridge: Once your hips are lifted in the bridge pose, extend one leg straight out for an added challenge.

- Bridge with Arm Movement: While in the bridge position, move your arms overhead and then back down to increase coordination.

- Static Bridge Hold: Lift into the bridge pose and hold the position for a longer duration, say 30 seconds to a minute.

- Pilates Bridge: It's a variation where you articulate your spine as you lift and lower, focusing on the movement of each vertebra.

SCAN the QR for the Video Bonus

FRONTAL HIP FLEXOR STRETCH

Description & Benefit: The Frontal Hip Flexor Stretch is a crucial exercise designed to target and elongate the hip flexor muscles, which are often shortened from long periods of sitting. Stretching these muscles can alleviate hip discomfort, improve posture, and promote better overall mobility. For seniors, this stretch is especially beneficial to counteract the effects of reduced activity, aiding in walking and reducing the risk of falls. Additionally, a flexible hip flexor can ease day-to-day tasks, from getting out of a chair to climbing stairs.

Instructions:

1. Begin by standing up straight with feet hip-width apart for stability.
2. Take a step back with your right foot and bend both knees to lower into a lunge. Ensure your left knee is aligned with your left ankle.
3. As you descend into the lunge, keep your torso upright and push your hips forward slightly. You should feel a stretch along the front of your right hip.
4. Hold the stretch for 20-30 seconds, keeping your shoulders relaxed and back.

5. Push off your back foot and return to the starting position.

6. Repeat the stretch on the left side.

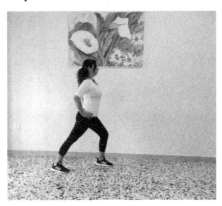

Tips:

- Keep your back straight and avoid leaning forward. This ensures the stretch targets the hip flexors accurately.

- If balance is a concern, perform this stretch near a wall or sturdy surface to hold onto.

- Engage your abdominal muscles during the stretch for stability and to protect the lower back.

- Breathe deeply and consistently throughout the stretch, aiding muscle relaxation.

Alternative exercises:

- Seated Hip Flexor Stretch: Sit on the edge of a sturdy chair. Extend one leg back, keeping both hips facing forward. Lean slightly forward to intensify the stretch.

- Quadriceps Stretch: While standing, bend one knee, bringing your heel toward your buttock. Hold your ankle and gently pull closer to your body.

- Butterfly Stretch: Sit on the ground, bring the soles of your feet together, and gently press your knees towards the floor.

- Psoas Stretch: Lying on your back, pull one knee to your chest, allowing the opposite leg to stretch out straight on the ground.

34

SIDE CLAMSHELL MOVEMENT

Description & Benefit: The Side Clamshell Movement is a popular exercise that targets the muscles of the outer thigh and buttocks, specifically the gluteus medius. This muscle is essential for hip stabilization, which in turn, plays a pivotal role in walking, standing, and balancing. For seniors, strengthening these areas can lead to improved posture, reduced risk of hip injuries, and enhanced overall mobility. Regularly practicing the clamshell exercise can also alleviate pain related to weak hip muscles.

Instructions:

1. Begin by lying on your side with your legs stacked on top of each other and knees bent at a 90-degree angle. Rest your head on your lower arm or use your hand as a pillow.
2. Keeping your feet touching each other, raise the upper knee as high as possible without moving your lower leg or rolling your back. Your legs should resemble a clamshell opening.
3. Pause at the top for a moment, feeling the squeeze in your outer hip.
4. Slowly lower the knee back to the starting position to complete one repetition.
5. Perform the desired number of repetitions on one side before switching to the other.

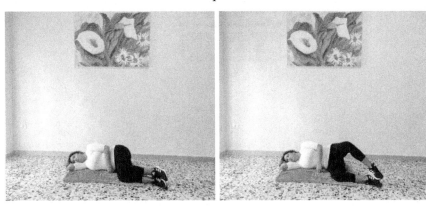

Tips:

- Ensure that your hips remain stacked throughout the movement. Avoid rolling back or forward.
- Engage your core muscles during the exercise to maintain stability and enhance the effectiveness of the movement.
- To increase resistance and further challenge your muscles, consider using a resistance band wrapped around your thighs.
- Focus on the quality of the movement rather than the quantity. It's essential to maintain proper form throughout.

Alternative exercises:

- Fire Hydrants: Start on all fours in a tabletop position. Keeping the knee bent, lift one leg out to the side and then return it to the starting position.

- Hip Bridges: Lie on your back with knees bent and feet flat on the floor. Lift your hips off the ground, squeezing the glutes at the top, then lower back down.

- Lateral Leg Raises: Lying on your side, straighten both legs. Lift the top leg up to about 45 degrees, then lower it back down.

- Standing Leg Lifts: Stand beside a wall or chair for support. Keeping your leg straight, lift it out to the side and then return to the starting position.

SCAN the QR for the Video Bonus

3.2 Lengthening the Legs

SEATED HAMSTRING REACH

Description & Benefit: The Seated Hamstring Reach focuses primarily on stretching and lengthening the hamstring muscles located at the back of the thigh. These muscles play a crucial role in activities like walking, bending, and sitting. As we age, our hamstrings can become tight and less flexible, which can lead to discomfort, reduced mobility, and a heightened risk of injuries. Regularly practicing the Seated Hamstring Reach can help maintain flexibility, improve posture, reduce lower back pain, and enhance overall leg function.

Instructions:

1. Start by sitting on the edge of a sturdy chair with your feet flat on the ground and legs hip-width apart.
2. Extend one leg straight out in front of you with the heel touching the ground and toes pointing upwards.
3. Keeping your back straight, hinge at the hips and lean forward gently until you feel a comfortable stretch at the back of your extended leg.
4. Reach both hands towards the toes of the extended leg, holding for 15-30 seconds.
5. Slowly return to the starting position and repeat with the other leg.

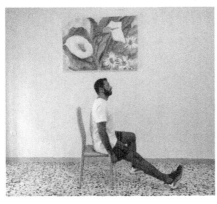 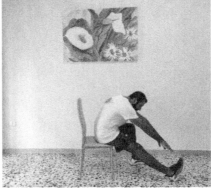

Tips:

- It's essential to keep your back straight and not rounded during the exercise. This ensures that the stretch targets the hamstrings rather than putting strain on the back.
- Always stretch to the point of tension but not pain. If you feel any sharp pain, ease off a bit.

- Take deep, slow breaths during the stretch to help your muscles relax and increase flexibility.
- For enhanced stability, ensure that the foot of your bent leg is firmly planted on the ground.

Alternative exercises:

- Standing Hamstring Stretch: Stand upright and place one heel on a slightly raised surface. Keeping both legs straight, hinge forward from the hips.
- Lying Hamstring Stretch with a Strap: Lie flat on your back and wrap a strap or towel around the ball of one foot. Gently pull the strap towards you, straightening the leg until a stretch is felt.
- Forward Bend: Stand with feet hip-width apart and slowly bend forward from the hips, reaching towards the ground or as far as comfortable.
- Wall Hamstring Stretch: Lie on the ground close to a wall and raise one leg, resting it against the wall while the other remains flat on the ground. Adjust the distance from the wall to increase or decrease the stretch intensity.

SCAN the QR for the Video Bonus

BALANCED QUAD PULL

Description & Benefit: The Balanced Quad Pull is a powerful exercise designed to stretch the quadriceps—the group of muscles located at the front of the thigh. These muscles are essential for actions like walking, running, and climbing stairs. Over time, especially with decreased activity, the quadriceps can become tight, limiting mobility and increasing the risk of strains. Regularly performing the Balanced Quad Pull can enhance flexibility, improve balance, reduce the risk of injuries, and support better posture.

Instructions:

1. Begin by standing next to a wall or a sturdy piece of furniture for support.
2. Shift your weight onto one leg.
3. With your free hand, gently grasp the ankle of the opposite leg.

4. Pull your heel towards your buttocks, ensuring that your knees are close together and your torso remains upright.

5. Hold the stretch for 15-30 seconds, feeling a stretch along the front of your thigh.

6. Slowly release and switch to the other leg.

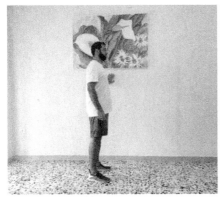 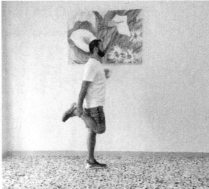

Tips:

- Keep your abdominal muscles engaged and maintain an upright posture throughout the stretch to prevent arching your back.

- If you experience any pain or discomfort in the knee, adjust your grip or reduce the intensity of the pull.

- Focus on your breathing. Deep, slow breaths can facilitate a deeper stretch and help with relaxation.

- For an added balance challenge, try performing the stretch without holding onto any support, but always prioritize safety.

Alternative exercises:

- Lying Quad Stretch: Lie on your side and pull your top leg's heel towards your buttocks. Use a strap or towel if you can't reach your ankle.

- Lunges: Step forward with one foot and lower your body until both knees are bent at a 90-degree angle. The back knee should hover just above the ground. This not only stretches the quadriceps but also works on strengthening them.

- Foam Roller Quad Stretch: Position a foam roller under your thighs while lying face down, and roll slowly from the hips to the knees.

- Pigeon Pose: This yoga pose stretches both the quadriceps of the back leg and the glutes of the front leg. Start in a plank position, bring one leg forward, and let it rest on the ground in front of you while extending the other leg behind.

SCAN the QR for the Video Bonus

BUTTERFLY INNER THIGH STRETCH

Description & Benefit: The Butterfly Inner Thigh Stretch is a classic seated exercise targeting the adductor muscles found along the inner thigh. These muscles play a crucial role in hip stabilization and leg movements, such as walking or turning. Tightness in this area can lead to imbalances, affecting gait and posture. Regularly incorporating the Butterfly Stretch can increase inner thigh flexibility, alleviate muscle tightness, and reduce the risk of related strains.

Instructions:

1. Begin by sitting on the floor with a straight spine.
2. Bend your knees outward and place the soles of your feet together, bringing them as close to your pelvis as comfortably possible.
3. Hold onto your ankles or toes with your hands.
4. Gently press your knees toward the floor using your elbows. Aim for a gentle stretch along your inner thighs.
5. Hold this position for 20-30 seconds, then slowly release.

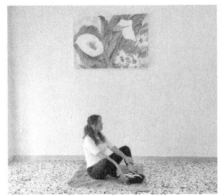 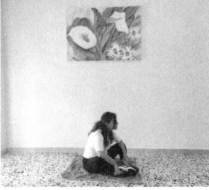

Tips:

- Ensure your back remains straight during the exercise. If you find yourself rounding your back, sit on a cushion or block to elevate your hips.
- Breathe deeply throughout the stretch, allowing each exhale to deepen the stretch slightly.
- Do not force your knees down. Apply gentle pressure for a comfortable stretch.
- To intensify the stretch, lean your upper body slightly forward while maintaining a straight back.

Alternative exercises:

- Wide-legged Forward Bend: From a standing position, spread your legs wide apart. With a straight back, hinge at the hips and fold forward, reaching your hands towards the ground.
- Side Lunge: Start with feet together. Step one foot out to the side, bending the knee into a lunge while keeping the other leg straight. Feel the stretch along the inner thigh of the straight leg.
- Leg Swings: Holding onto a support, swing one leg side to side in front of the other. This dynamic stretch can help warm up the inner thigh muscles.
- Frog Pose: Start on all fours, then widen your knees until a stretch is felt in the inner thighs. Keep your feet pointing outwards and rest on your forearms for a deeper stretch.

DYNAMIC CALF ELEVATIONS

Description & Benefit: Dynamic Calf Elevations are an effective exercise to engage and strengthen the calf muscles, which are pivotal in activities like walking, running, and jumping. As the calf muscles are frequently utilized, they can become tight or fatigued. This exercise not only enhances muscle tone but also promotes flexibility and circulation in the lower legs, reducing the risk of injuries like calf strains or Achilles tendinitis.

Instructions:

1. Begin by standing upright with feet hip-width apart.
2. Engage your core for stability.
3. Slowly rise onto your tiptoes, lifting your heels as high as possible.
4. Pause momentarily at the top of the elevation.
5. Gradually lower your heels back to the floor.
6. Repeat the motion for 10-15 repetitions, ensuring a smooth and controlled movement throughout.

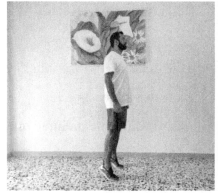 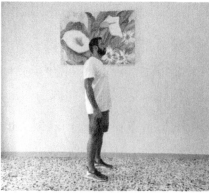

Tips:

- Ensure you're pressing evenly through the balls of both feet while rising to prevent any imbalances.

- For added stability or to intensify the exercise, perform this near a wall or counter, lightly resting one hand on it.

- As you progress, consider adding resistance by holding dumbbells in your hands or wearing a weighted vest.

- Focus on the quality of each elevation rather than the quantity. It's more beneficial to perform fewer repetitions with good form.

Alternative exercises:

- Seated Calf Raise: Sit on a bench or chair with feet flat on the ground. Lift your heels off the ground while keeping your toes on the floor. This targets the soleus muscle in the calf.

- Bent-Knee Calf Raise: Similar to the standard calf raise but with a slight bend in the knees, which engages different parts of the calf muscles.

- Single Leg Calf Raise: Elevate one foot off the ground, performing the raise using only the other leg. This increases the intensity as one leg bears all the weight.

- Jumping Jacks: This classic exercise also engages the calves, especially when emphasis is placed on springing from the toes during each jump.

SCAN the QR for the Video Bonus

GROUND-TOUCH FORWARD BEND

Description & Benefit: The Ground-Touch Forward Bend, often simply known as the Forward Bend, is a stretching exercise that targets the hamstrings, calves, and lower back. It aids in increasing flexibility in the posterior chain, which can significantly benefit daily movements and posture. By performing this stretch regularly, individuals can reduce tension in the lower back, enhance circulation, and alleviate tightness in the legs.

Instructions:

1. Begin in a standing position with your feet hip-width apart and arms resting by your sides.
2. Inhale deeply and extend your arms overhead, lengthening the spine.
3. Exhale as you hinge at the hips, folding forward towards the ground. Aim to keep your spine straight and long.
4. Allow your hands to reach towards the ground. If you can, touch the ground or your toes. If not, simply let your arms hang or grasp your elbows.
5. Keep your knees slightly bent to avoid straining the hamstrings.
6. Hold the position for 20-30 seconds, breathing deeply.
7. To come out of the bend, inhale and slowly roll up, vertebra by vertebra, until you're standing upright again.

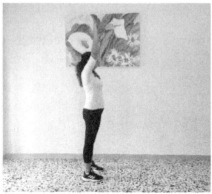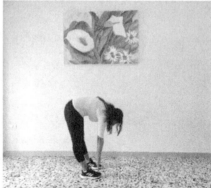

Tips:

- Ensure that the bend originates from the hips, not the waist. This keeps the spine protected and maximizes the stretch in the hamstrings.
- If you find it challenging to touch the ground, consider using a yoga block or similar prop to bridge the gap.
- Engage your core throughout the exercise to provide additional support to the back.

44

- Avoid locking your knees completely; maintaining a micro-bend helps in preventing any undue stress on the joints.

Alternative exercises:

- Halfway Lift (Ardha Uttanasana): From the forward bend position, raise your torso so it's parallel to the ground and your hands rest on your shins. This gives a milder stretch to the hamstrings and lower back.

- Seated Forward Bend (Paschimottanasana): Sit with legs extended straight. Hinge at the hips to fold forward, reaching your hands toward your feet.

- Standing Calf Stretch: Place your hands on a wall, extend one leg straight back, pressing the heel into the ground. This isolates the stretch more to the calf.

- Wide-Legged Forward Bend: Stand with feet wider than hip-width, hinge at the hips, and fold forward. This variation can be easier on the back and also stretches the inner thighs.

SCAN the QR for the Video Bonus

45

3.3 Ankle and Foot Flexibility

ROTATIONAL ANKLE CIRCLES

Description & Benefit: Rotational Ankle Circles are a simple yet effective exercise to enhance the flexibility and mobility of the ankle joint. By performing this movement, seniors can improve circulation in the feet, reduce stiffness, and potentially decrease the risk of ankle injuries. This exercise aids in lubricating the ankle joint, making daily activities like walking and stair climbing smoother and more comfortable.

Instructions:

1. Begin by sitting in a comfortable chair with your feet flat on the ground.
2. Extend one leg out in front of you, keeping the knee slightly bent.
3. Point your toes and start making circles with your foot, moving only from the ankle joint.
4. Complete 10-15 rotations in a clockwise direction.
5. Switch to counter-clockwise and perform another 10-15 rotations.
6. Lower the foot back to the ground and repeat with the opposite ankle.

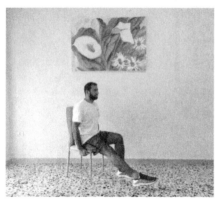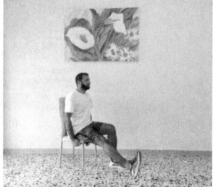

Tips:

- Ensure the movement is isolated to the ankle, avoiding movement in the leg.
- Perform the exercise slowly, focusing on the full range of motion rather than speed.
- If you feel any sharp pain, stop the exercise and consider consulting a professional.
- As you progress, try performing the exercise while standing, holding onto a chair or wall for balance.

Alternative exercises:

- Toe Tapping: While seated, keep your heels on the ground and tap your toes repeatedly. This exercise activates the shin muscles and enhances foot mobility.

- Heel Raises: Stand tall and lift your heels, balancing on the balls of your feet. This strengthens the calf muscles and enhances ankle stability.

- Ankle Flex and Point: Extend your leg and alternate between pointing your toes and flexing the foot upwards. This simple motion stretches both the shin and calf muscles.

- Ankle Alphabet: Pretend your big toe is a pen and "write" the alphabet in the air. This exercise provides a broader range of motion than simple circles.

SCAN the QR for the Video Bonus

RHYTHMIC TOE TAPS

Description & Benefit: Rhythmic Toe Taps are a straightforward yet effective exercise designed to boost the agility and strength of the foot muscles. By incorporating this activity, seniors can enhance their foot coordination, leading to improved balance and a reduced risk of trips and falls. Regularly performing toe taps can also increase blood circulation in the feet, which can be beneficial for those who experience foot cramps or swelling.

Instructions:

1. Begin seated in a sturdy chair, keeping your back straight and feet flat on the floor.
2. Starting with your right foot, lift the toes while keeping the heel anchored to the ground.
3. Tap the toes back down in a rhythmic motion.
4. Continue tapping for a count of 15-20 times.
5. Switch to your left foot and repeat the tapping process.
6. For added challenge, try performing the taps at different speeds.

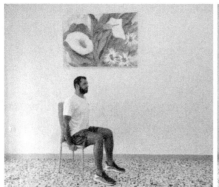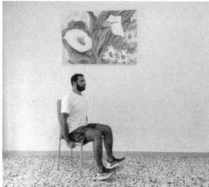

Tips:

- Ensure you're lifting your toes as high as comfortably possible to maximize the exercise's benefits.

- Focus on maintaining a rhythmic motion, which can enhance foot coordination.

- If you experience any pain or discomfort, slow down or stop the exercise.

- Over time, as your strength and agility improve, increase the count or duration of the taps.

Alternative exercises:

- Heel Taps: Similar to toe taps but lift your heels while keeping the balls of your feet on the ground. This targets the shin muscles.

- Side-to-Side Foot Taps: Start with both feet together. Tap the right foot to the side and then return to the starting position. Repeat with the left foot. This aids in lateral foot strength and coordination.

- Marching in Place: While seated, lift one knee at a time as if you're marching. This engages both the legs and feet and improves overall coordination.

- Ankle Pumps: With your foot flat on the ground, push down with your toes then lift them up, alternating in a pumping motion. This exercise enhances calf and shin strength and boosts circulation in the ankle area.

48

DUAL-DIRECTION FOOT FLEXES

Description & Benefit: Dual-Direction Foot Flexes focus on enhancing the flexibility and strength of the foot and ankle muscles. This exercise plays a pivotal role in promoting good foot health, as it works both the dorsiflexors (top of the foot) and the plantar flexors (bottom of the foot). Regular practice can lead to improved balance, a decreased risk of foot-related injuries, and better support for walking and other daily activities.

Instructions:

1. Start by sitting comfortably in a sturdy chair, ensuring that both feet are flat on the ground.
2. Lift your right foot slightly off the floor.
3. Begin by pointing your toes away from you, flexing your foot in a downward direction. This is the plantar flexion.
4. Now, pull your toes towards you, flexing your foot upwards. This is the dorsiflexion.
5. Alternate between these two flexes for a count of 10-15 times.
6. Set the right foot down and repeat the process with the left foot.

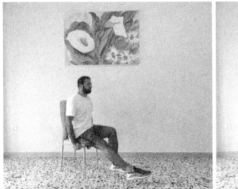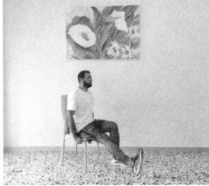

Tips:

- Aim for a full range of motion, ensuring you're pointing and flexing as far as your foot comfortably allows.
- Maintain a slow and controlled movement to avoid straining the foot muscles.
- Always keep your ankle relaxed, allowing the foot's motion to stem mainly from the ankle joint.
- If you notice any discomfort or pain, ease up on the intensity or pause the exercise.

49

Alternative exercises:

- Ankle Circles: Lift one foot and make circles with the toes, rotating the ankle. This enhances joint flexibility and can help relieve stiffness.

- Toe Tapping: While keeping your heels on the ground, lift and tap your toes rhythmically. This targets the dorsiflexor muscles.

- Heel Raises: With feet flat on the ground, lift the heels, pressing the balls of the feet into the floor. This strengthens the calf and the plantar flexor muscles.

- Towel Scrunches: Place a towel on the floor and, using your toes, try to scrunch it towards you. This is great for strengthening and increasing dexterity in the toes.

HEEL-FOCUSED WALKING

Description & Benefit: Heel-Focused Walking, often referred to as "heel-to-toe walking," is a targeted exercise that enhances balance, coordination, and the strength of the foot and lower leg muscles. By emphasizing the heel strike and rolling onto the toes, this exercise not only supports better walking mechanics but also aids in the prevention of foot-related issues and injuries.

Instructions:

1. Begin by standing upright with your feet hip-width apart.
2. Take a step forward, emphasizing the heel strike first.
3. Slowly roll from the heel, through the arch, and then onto the ball of your foot, finishing the step on your toes.
4. Continue walking in this manner, focusing on the heel-to-toe motion with each step.
5. Aim to walk for at least 20-30 steps in one direction, then turn around and walk back to your starting point.

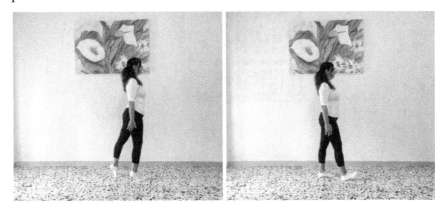

Tips:

- Maintain a straight and aligned posture throughout the exercise. Keep your head up and shoulders relaxed.
- Initially, it might be beneficial to practice this exercise near a wall or with a supportive handrail to ensure balance.
- As you progress, try to challenge your balance by walking along a straight line or practicing on different surfaces.
- Focus on a smooth rolling motion through the foot, ensuring each part of the foot touches the ground sequentially.

Alternative exercises:

- Toe-Focused Walking: Emphasize walking on the balls of your feet without letting heels touch the ground. This strengthens the calves and challenges balance.

- Sideways Walking: Walk side-to-side, which engages different muscles and enhances lateral movement coordination.

- Walking on Uneven Surfaces: Walk on grass, sand, or gravel to challenge foot strength and balance.

- Backward Walking: Walking backward not only requires coordination but also activates different muscle groups and can improve proprioception. Always ensure the path behind is clear and safe.

SCAN the QR for the Video Bonus

Chapter 4: Core and Balance Stretches for Seniors

4.1 Abdominal Stretches

EXTENDED COBRA POSE

Description & Benefit: The Extended Cobra Pose, an adaptation of the traditional Cobra Pose, offers a gentle backbend that primarily focuses on the abdominal muscles. This pose helps in strengthening the spine, relieving back pain, and promoting better posture. It also helps in opening the chest and shoulders, thus enhancing lung capacity.

Instructions:

1. Begin by lying face down on a mat with your legs extended behind you. Keep your feet hip-width apart and press the tops of your feet into the mat.
2. Place your hands underneath your shoulders with your fingers pointing forward.
3. Inhale deeply, and as you exhale, gently lift your head and chest off the ground using the strength of your back muscles. Make sure your pubic bone remains in contact with the mat.
4. Slide your shoulder blades down your back and squeeze your elbows towards your body.
5. Hold the pose for 15-30 seconds, breathing evenly.
6. To release, exhale and gently lower your chest and head back to the mat.

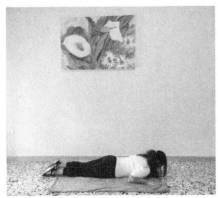 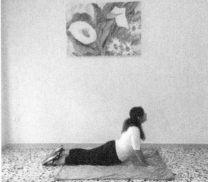

Tips:

- Keep your elbows close to your body throughout the pose to avoid straining your shoulders.

53

- Ensure you lift using your back muscles and not by pressing too much through your hands.
- If you feel any strain in your lower back, reduce the height of your lift.
- Engage your abdominal muscles to support your spine.

Alternative exercises:
- Baby Cobra Pose: A milder version where you lift your chest only slightly off the ground.
- Sphinx Pose: Elevate your upper torso by resting on your forearms.
- Bow Pose: Offers a deeper backbend, but may not be suitable for everyone.
- Bridge Pose: A backbend that also targets the legs and glutes.

SEATED FORWARD BEND

Description & Benefit: The Seated Forward Bend is a fundamental stretch that promotes flexibility and relaxation. For seniors, this exercise is particularly beneficial as it stretches the spine, shoulders, hamstrings, and pelvis. Regularly practicing this bend can help alleviate stress, calm the mind, and improve digestion. Additionally, it aids in reducing fatigue, headaches, and anxiety.

Instructions:

1. Start by sitting on a mat with your legs extended straight in front of you. Ensure your spine is upright and your feet are flexed towards you.
2. Inhale deeply, extending your arms overhead and lengthening your spine.
3. As you exhale, hinge at your hips to lean forward, aiming to bring your chest towards your knees. Extend your arms out to grasp your feet, ankles, or shins, depending on your flexibility level.
4. Keep your back as straight as possible, aiming to get your chest to your thighs rather than trying to get your head to your knees.
5. Hold this position for 20-30 seconds, taking deep and even breaths.
6. To release, inhale and slowly lift your torso back to the starting position.

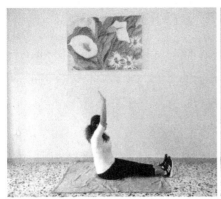 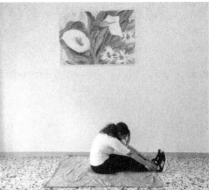

Tips:

- Ensure you are bending from the hips and not rounding the spine. Imagine your torso as a hinge that's folding forward.

- If you cannot reach your feet, consider using a strap or a towel around the soles of your feet for support.

- Avoid forcing the stretch. Go to the point where you feel a mild tension, not pain.

Alternative exercises:

- Supported Forward Bend: Use a cushion or a folded blanket under your sit bones for better support and alignment.

- Standing Forward Bend: A standing version of the stretch which also engages the leg muscles more.

- Wide-legged Seated Forward Bend: Sit with your legs wide apart and bend forward, targeting the inner thighs.

- Paschimottanasana with Chair: For those with limited mobility, use a chair to rest your arms and head while bending forward. This ensures less strain on the back.

SCAN the QR for the Video Bonus

MODIFIED BOAT POSE

Description & Benefit: The Modified Boat Pose, a gentler variation of the traditional Boat Pose (Navasana), focuses on strengthening the core and hip flexors without straining the back. Particularly for seniors, maintaining core strength is vital for overall stability, balance, and daily activities. This pose not only tones the abdominal muscles but also stimulates the kidneys, thyroid, and intestines, aiding in digestion.

Instructions:

1. Begin by sitting on a mat with your knees bent and feet flat on the floor. Ensure your spine is elongated and your chest is open.
2. Place your hands behind your thighs, just below the knees. Lean back slightly, lifting your feet off the ground until your shins are parallel to the floor.
3. Balance on your sit bones, keeping your spine straight. Engage your core muscles.
4. Extend your arms forward, parallel to the ground, palms facing each other.
5. Hold the pose for 5-10 breaths, keeping your chest lifted and spine straight.
6. To release, gently lower your feet back to the floor and relax your arms.

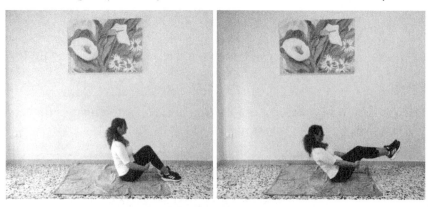

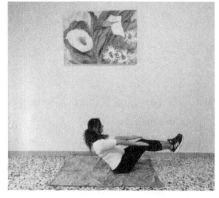

Tips:

- Keep your shoulders relaxed and down, away from the ears.

- If you feel strain in the neck or lower back, ensure you're engaging your core muscles adequately and not arching your back.
- Focus on your breathing, taking deep and even breaths throughout the pose.

Alternative exercises:

- Full Boat Pose: For those with more core strength, extend the legs straight, forming a 'V' shape with the body.
- Low Boat Pose: From the Full Boat Pose, lower the upper and lower body towards the ground without letting them touch the floor. This intensifies the abdominal engagement.
- Boat Pose with a Strap: Use a yoga strap or a belt around the soles of your feet, holding its ends in your hands, for added stability and support.
- Half Boat Pose with Bent Knees: Keep the knees bent while lifting the feet, making it easier to hold the pose.

GENTLE CORE TWIST

Description & Benefit: The Gentle Core Twist is a seated exercise that targets the oblique muscles, helping to improve rotational mobility in the torso and strengthening the core. For seniors, maintaining a strong core is crucial for balance, posture, and functional movements in daily life. This twist also aids in massaging internal organs, improving digestion, and facilitating detoxification.

Instructions:

1. Begin by sitting tall on a sturdy chair, feet flat on the ground, hip-width apart.
2. Place your hands on your shoulders, elbows pointing out to the sides.
3. Keeping your hips and legs stationary, gently rotate your upper body to the right, aiming to get your left elbow pointing forward and your right elbow pointing backward.
4. Hold this twist for 3-5 breaths, feeling the stretch in your obliques and spine.
5. Slowly return to the center, then repeat the twist on the left side.
6. Complete this rotation 3-5 times on each side.

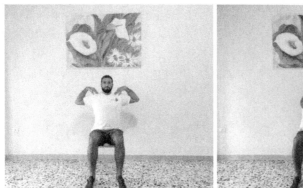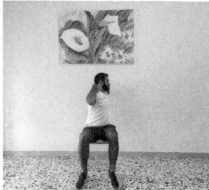

Tips:

- Ensure your spine remains straight throughout the twist. Think of elongating your spine as you rotate.

- Move with your breath. Inhale as you come to the center, and exhale as you twist.

- Do not force the twist. Rotate only as far as it feels comfortable without straining.

- Keep your feet firmly grounded, ensuring your lower body remains stable.

Alternative exercises:

- Standing Core Twist: Stand with feet hip-width apart, hands on shoulders, and perform the twist while standing.

- Extended Arm Core Twist: Instead of placing hands on shoulders, extend your arms out to the sides at shoulder height and perform the twist.

- Core Twist with Resistance Band: Hold a resistance band with both hands, arms extended in front of you, and twist, pulling the band to one side.

- Lying Core Twist: Lie on your back on a mat, knees bent, arms extended to the sides. Drop your knees to one side, keeping shoulders on the ground, and then return to center and drop knees to the other side.

SCAN the QR for the Video Bonus

4.2 Oblique and Lower Back Stretches

SEATED SIDE BEND

Description & Benefit: The Seated Side Bend is an effective stretch targeting the oblique muscles, the muscles running along the side of the torso. This exercise enhances lateral mobility of the spine, improves posture, and aids in reducing stiffness in the midsection. It also helps in elongating the side muscles, which can alleviate discomfort or tightness, especially for seniors who spend long periods sitting or have limited movement throughout the day.

Instructions:

1. Begin by sitting on a sturdy chair with your feet flat on the ground, hip-width apart.
2. Keep your spine straight, arms resting by your sides.
3. Inhale deeply as you extend your right arm upwards towards the ceiling.
4. Exhale and gently bend to the left side, feeling a stretch along the right side of your torso. Your left hand can slide down the side of the chair for added support.
5. Hold the side bend for 3-5 breaths, feeling the stretch intensify with each exhale.
6. Inhale as you return to the center, lowering your right arm.
7. Repeat the bend on the other side with the left arm raised.
8. Complete 3-5 repetitions on each side.

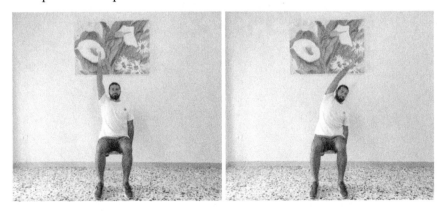

Tips:

- Ensure you are bending from the waist and not the hips. Imagine your torso between two panes of glass, moving only to the side and not forward or backward.
- Keep both hips firmly grounded on the chair, ensuring even weight distribution.

- To deepen the stretch, you can extend both arms overhead, holding the wrist of the bending side with the opposite hand.
- Focus on elongating the spine as you bend, rather than trying to bend too far.

Alternative exercises:

- Standing Side Bend: Perform the same side bend, but from a standing position. This variation can challenge balance and engage the leg muscles.
- Extended Leg Side Bend: While seated, extend the opposite leg of the bending side outward and bend towards the extended leg.
- Side Bend with a Resistance Band: Hold a resistance band overhead with both hands, shoulder-width apart. Bend to one side, keeping tension in the band.
- Dynamic Side Bend: Instead of holding the bend, move fluidly from one side to the other, creating a waving motion with the spine. This can help increase flexibility and warmth in the core region.

SCAN the QR for the Video Bonus

SUPINE KNEE TWIST

Description & Benefit: The Supine Knee Twist is a gentle yet effective stretch targeting the lower back, obliques, and hips. By allowing the spine to rotate in a controlled manner, this exercise helps in releasing tension in the lower back, enhancing spinal flexibility, and promoting better hip mobility. Regular practice can lead to improved posture, reduced back discomfort, and increased overall mobility, especially crucial for seniors.

Instructions:

1. Start by lying flat on your back on a comfortable mat or carpeted surface. Extend your arms outward in a 'T' shape for stability.
2. Bend your knees, keeping your feet flat on the ground.
3. While keeping your shoulders pressed firmly against the floor, gently lower both bent knees to one side, aiming to get them as close to the ground as possible.
4. Turn your head to the opposite direction for an added neck stretch.
5. Hold the twist for 15-30 seconds, breathing deeply and feeling the stretch across your lower back and side.
6. Gently return your knees to the center and repeat the twist on the other side.
7. Perform 2-3 repetitions on each side.

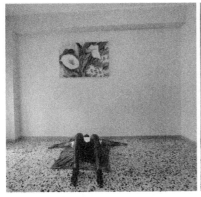 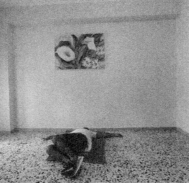

Tips:

- Engage your core muscles to support your lower back throughout the exercise.
- Keep both shoulders flat on the ground, resisting the urge to lift the opposite shoulder as you twist.
- Move slowly and deliberately, ensuring you never force your knees further than your comfort level.

61

- If needed, place a cushion or folded blanket between your knees for added comfort.

Alternative exercises:

- Leg Extended Supine Twist: Instead of keeping knees bent, extend the top leg straight out as you twist, providing a deeper stretch for the hamstrings and IT band.
- Seated Chair Twist: Sit on a chair, cross one leg over the other, and gently twist towards the crossed leg, using the chair's backrest for leverage.
- Cat-Cow Twist: Start in a tabletop position, as you arch your back (cow pose), twist slightly to one side, then round the back (cat pose) and twist to the other side.
- Lunging Twist: Begin in a lunge position with one foot forward. Place the opposite hand on the ground and twist, extending the other arm toward the ceiling. This stretches the hip flexors while incorporating a spinal twist.

CAT-COW STRETCH VARIATION

Description & Benefit: The Cat-Cow Stretch Variation is a modified version of the traditional yoga Cat-Cow pose, tailored specifically for seniors. This movement aids in enhancing spinal flexibility, relieving tension in the neck and back, and promoting better posture. Regular practice can stimulate and strengthen the spine, helping to alleviate general back discomfort and tightness.

Instructions:

1. Start by sitting comfortably on a chair with your feet flat on the ground, hip-width apart, and hands resting on your knees.
2. Inhale deeply. As you exhale, arch your back, pushing your chest forward and looking up towards the ceiling. This is the "Cow" position.
3. Inhale again. As you exhale, round your back, tuck your chin to your chest, and push your mid-back towards the chair. This is the "Cat" position.
4. Continue to move fluidly between the two positions, synchronizing your movements with your breath.
5. Perform this cycle for 5-10 repetitions.

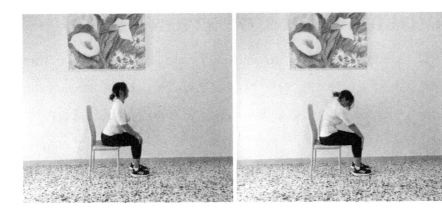

Tips:

- Ensure your movements are slow and controlled. Avoid any jerky motions.
- Syncing your breath with the movements enhances the stretch and helps in relaxation.
- Keep your shoulders relaxed and away from your ears throughout the stretch.
- If you have any neck issues, keep the neck neutral rather than flexing and extending it.

Alternative exercises:

- Traditional Cat-Cow Pose: This is done on hands and knees on the floor, moving between arching and rounding the back.
- Seated Spinal Twist: Sitting on a chair, hold the backrest with one hand and gently twist towards that side.
- Child's Pose Variation: Sit back on your heels (or use cushions for comfort), stretch arms forward on the ground, and gently sway side to side to stretch the sides of the torso.
- Seated Forward Bend: Sitting on the edge of a chair, extend your legs and hinge at the hips to lean forward, reaching hands towards the feet. This stretches the back and hamstrings.

CHILD'S POSE SIDE STRETCH

Description & Benefit: The Child's Pose Side Stretch is an enhanced version of the traditional yoga Child's Pose, with an added side stretch to target the oblique muscles and the sides of the torso. This variation provides a deeper stretch, promoting flexibility along the spine's lateral aspects and helping to alleviate tightness in the sides of the back. It's an excellent stretch for seniors looking to improve their side flexibility and maintain a supple spine.

Instructions:

1. Begin by kneeling on a soft surface, such as a yoga mat or carpet, with your big toes touching and knees spread apart.
2. Sit back onto your heels, keeping your arms extended in front of you.
3. Walk both hands over to the right side, stretching the left side of your body. Your left hip should remain over your left heel.
4. Lower your forehead towards the ground and feel the stretch along the left side of your torso.
5. Hold for a few breaths, then walk your hands back to the center and over to the left side, repeating the stretch for the right side of your body.
6. After stretching both sides, return to the center and sit back up.

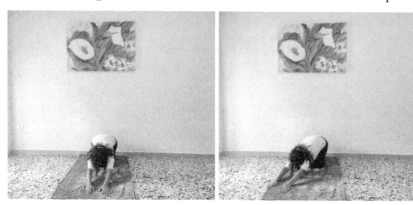

Tips:

- Breathe deeply and evenly throughout the stretch, focusing on expanding the rib cage.
- Ensure you're stretching the side of the body rather than leaning forward or backward.
- Use a cushion or folded blanket under your knees for added comfort if needed.
- Listen to your body and don't push yourself too hard. It's essential to remain comfortable and avoid pain.

Alternative exercises:

- Traditional Child's Pose: Sit back on your heels, extend your arms forward, and rest your forehead on the ground.

- Extended Puppy Pose: Start on all fours, keep your hips over your knees, and walk your hands forward, lowering your chest towards the ground.

- Seated Side Bend: While seated, extend one arm overhead and lean to the opposite side, stretching the side of the torso.

- Standing Side Stretch: Stand tall, clasp your hands overhead, and lean to one side, stretching the side body.

SCAN the QR for the Video Bonus

Chapter 5: 4-Week Stretching Plan

Imagine our stretching routines as stepping stones on a serene garden path. You begin with the beginner's stone, with gentle and welcoming steps laid out for you. As you gain strength and confidence, the intermediate stones beckon. They offer a slightly brisker pace but remain comfortably spaced. And when you feel ready, the advanced stones present an invigorating challenge, drawing upon all you've learned.

However, this garden path has no rush. You're encouraged to spend as much time as you need on each stone, embracing steady progression and finding a pace that feels just right. Remember, consistency is the guiding light on this journey, so even small steps, when taken regularly, can illuminate your way.

And always keep in mind: on any journey, it's wise to seek guidance from those familiar with the path. If ever in doubt, consulting a health professional can provide clarity and reassurance.

May your stretching journey be both invigorating and joyful as you continue reading and practicing.

5.1 Beginners Plan

Week 1

Day	Upper Body	Lower Body	Core & Balance
Mon	NECK TILTS (5m), SHOULDER ROLLS (5m)	GENTLE PIGEON POSE (5m), CHAIR-BASED HIP OPENER (5m)	SEATED TWIST STRETCH (10m)
Tue	NECK ROTATION (5m), TRICEP STRETCH (5m)	UPLIFTING BRIDGES (5m), BALANCED QUAD PULL (5m)	CAT-COW STRETCH (10m)
Wed	SHOULDER SHRUG STRETCH (5m), WRIST FLEXOR STRETCH (5m)	SEATED HAMSTRING REACH (5m), BUTTERFLY INNER THIGH STRETCH (5m)	CHILD'S POSE STRETCH (10m)
Thu	NECK TILTS (5m), WRIST EXTENSOR STRETCH (5m)	DYNAMIC CALF ELEVATIONS (5m), SIDE CLAMSHELL MOVEMENT (5m)	SEATED FORWARD BEND (10m)
Fri	SHOULDER ROLLS (5m), TRICEP STRETCH (5m)	GROUND-TOUCH FORWARD BEND (5m), GENTLE PIGEON POSE (5m)	GENTLE CORE TWIST (10m) .
Sat	NECK ROTATION (5m), WRIST FLEXOR STRETCH (5m)	CHAIR-BASED HIP OPENER (5m), UPLIFTING BRIDGES (5m)	CAT-COW STRETCH VARIATION (10m)
Sun	Rest	Rest	Rest

Week 2

Day	Upper Body	Lower Body	Core & Balance
Mon	SHOULDER ROLLS (5m), TRICEP STRETCH (5m)	GENTLE PIGEON POSE (5m), BALANCED QUAD PULL (5m)	SEATED TWIST STRETCH (10m)
Tue	NECK ROTATION (5m), WRIST FLEXOR STRETCH (5m)	UPLIFTING BRIDGES (5m), BUTTERFLY INNER THIGH STRETCH (5m)	CAT-COW STRETCH (10m)
Wed	NECK TILTS (5m), WRIST EXTENSOR STRETCH (5m)	DYNAMIC CALF ELEVATIONS (5m), SIDE CLAMSHELL MOVEMENT (5m)	CHILD'S POSE STRETCH (10m)
Thu	SHOULDER SHRUG STRETCH (5m), TRICEP STRETCH (5m)	CHAIR-BASED HIP OPENER (5m), SEATED HAMSTRING REACH (5m)	SEATED FORWARD BEND (10m)
Fri	NECK ROTATION (5m), SHOULDER ROLLS (5m)	GROUND-TOUCH FORWARD BEND (5m), GENTLE PIGEON POSE (5m)	GENTLE CORE TWIST (10m)
Sat	NECK TILTS (5m), WRIST FLEXOR STRETCH (5m)	UPLIFTING BRIDGES (5m), BALANCED QUAD PULL (5m)	CAT-COW STRETCH VARIATION (10m)
Sun	Rest	Rest	Rest

Week 3

Day	Upper Body	Lower Body	Core & Balance
Mon	SHOULDER ROLLS (5m), NECK TILTS (5m)	CHAIR-BASED HIP OPENER (5m), DYNAMIC CALF ELEVATIONS (5m)	SEATED TWIST STRETCH (10m)
Tue	TRICEP STRETCH (5m), WRIST FLEXOR STRETCH (5m)	UPLIFTING BRIDGES (5m), SIDE CLAMSHELL MOVEMENT (5m)	CAT-COW STRETCH (10m)
Wed	NECK ROTATION (5m), WRIST EXTENSOR STRETCH (5m)	BALANCED QUAD PULL (5m), GENTLE PIGEON POSE (5m)	CHILD'S POSE STRETCH (10m)
Thu	SHOULDER SHRUG STRETCH (5m), NECK TILTS (5m)	BUTTERFLY INNER THIGH STRETCH (5m), UPLIFTING BRIDGES (5m)	SEATED FORWARD BEND (10m)
Fri	SHOULDER ROLLS (5m), TRICEP STRETCH (5m)	GROUND-TOUCH FORWARD BEND (5m), CHAIR-BASED HIP OPENER (5m)	GENTLE CORE TWIST (10m)
Sat	NECK ROTATION (5m), WRIST FLEXOR STRETCH (5m)	DYNAMIC CALF ELEVATIONS (5m), BALANCED QUAD PULL (5m)	CAT-COW STRETCH VARIATION (10m)
Sun	Rest	Rest	Rest

Week 4

Day	Upper Body	Lower Body	Core & Balance
Mon	NECK TILTS (5m), SHOULDER ROLLS (5m)	GENTLE PIGEON POSE (5m), CHAIR-BASED HIP OPENER (5m)	SEATED TWIST STRETCH (10m)
Tue	NECK ROTATION (5m), TRICEP STRETCH (5m)	UPLIFTING BRIDGES (5m), BALANCED QUAD PULL (5m)	CAT-COW STRETCH (10m)
Wed	SHOULDER SHRUG STRETCH (5m), WRIST FLEXOR STRETCH (5m)	SEATED HAMSTRING REACH (5m), BUTTERFLY INNER THIGH STRETCH (5m)	CHILD'S POSE STRETCH (10m)
Thu	NECK TILTS (5m), WRIST EXTENSOR STRETCH (5m)	DYNAMIC CALF ELEVATIONS (5m), SIDE CLAMSHELL MOVEMENT (5m)	SEATED FORWARD BEND (10m)
Fri	SHOULDER ROLLS (5m), TRICEP STRETCH (5m)	GROUND-TOUCH FORWARD BEND (5m), GENTLE PIGEON POSE (5m)	GENTLE CORE TWIST (10m)
Sat	NECK ROTATION (5m), WRIST FLEXOR STRETCH (5m)	CHAIR-BASED HIP OPENER (5m), UPLIFTING BRIDGES (5m)	CAT-COW STRETCH VARIATION (10m)
Sun	Rest	Rest	Rest

5.2 Intermediate Plan

Week 1

Day	Upper Body	Lower Body	Core & Balance
Mon	NECK TILTS (5m), SHOULDER ROLLS (5m), NECK ROTATION (5m)	GENTLE PIGEON POSE (5m), CHAIR-BASED HIP OPENER (5m), UPLIFTING BRIDGES (5m)	SEATED TWIST STRETCH (5m), SEATED FORWARD BEND (5m)
Tue	TRICEP STRETCH (5m), WRIST FLEXOR STRETCH (5m), SHOULDER SHRUG STRETCH (5m)	BALANCED QUAD PULL (5m), SEATED HAMSTRING REACH (5m), BUTTERFLY INNER THIGH STRETCH (5m)	CAT-COW STRETCH (5m), GENTLE CORE TWIST (5m)
Wed	WRIST EXTENSOR STRETCH (5m), NECK TILTS (5m), SHOULDER ROLLS (5m)	DYNAMIC CALF ELEVATIONS (5m), GROUND-TOUCH FORWARD BEND (5m), SIDE CLAMSHELL MOVEMENT (5m)	CHILD'S POSE STRETCH (5m), MODIFIED BOAT POSE (5m)
Thu	NECK ROTATION (5m), TRICEP STRETCH (5m), WRIST FLEXOR STRETCH (5m)	CHAIR-BASED HIP OPENER (5m), UPLIFTING BRIDGES (5m), GENTLE PIGEON POSE (5m)	SEATED TWIST STRETCH (5m), EXTENDED COBRA POSE (5m)
Fri	SHOULDER SHRUG STRETCH (5m), WRIST EXTENSOR STRETCH (5m), NECK TILTS (5m)	BALANCED QUAD PULL (5m), SEATED HAMSTRING REACH (5m), DYNAMIC CALF ELEVATIONS (5m)	CAT-COW STRETCH VARIATION (5m), GENTLE CORE TWIST (5m)
Sat	SHOULDER ROLLS (5m), TRICEP STRETCH (5m), NECK ROTATION (5m)	BUTTERFLY INNER THIGH STRETCH (5m), GROUND-TOUCH FORWARD BEND (5m), SIDE CLAMSHELL MOVEMENT (5m)	CHILD'S POSE STRETCH (5m), SEATED FORWARD BEND (5m)
Sun	Rest	Rest	Rest

Week 2

Day	Upper Body	Lower Body	Core & Balance
Mon	NECK ROTATION (5m), TRICEP STRETCH (5m), WRIST FLEXOR STRETCH (5m)	UPLIFTING BRIDGES (5m), GENTLE PIGEON POSE (5m), BALANCED QUAD PULL (5m)	CAT-COW STRETCH (5m), MODIFIED BOAT POSE (5m)
Tue	SHOULDER ROLLS (5m), WRIST EXTENSOR STRETCH (5m), NECK TILTS (5m)	BUTTERFLY INNER THIGH STRETCH (5m), SEATED HAMSTRING REACH (5m), SIDE CLAMSHELL MOVEMENT (5m)	SEATED TWIST STRETCH (5m), GENTLE CORE TWIST (5m)
Wed	SHOULDER SHRUG STRETCH (5m), NECK ROTATION (5m), TRICEP STRETCH (5m)	DYNAMIC CALF ELEVATIONS (5m), GROUND-TOUCH FORWARD BEND (5m), CHAIR-BASED HIP OPENER (5m)	CHILD'S POSE STRETCH (5m), EXTENDED COBRA POSE (5m)
Thu	WRIST FLEXOR STRETCH (5m), NECK TILTS (5m), WRIST EXTENSOR STRETCH (5m)	GENTLE PIGEON POSE (5m), BALANCED QUAD PULL (5m), UPLIFTING BRIDGES (5m)	SEATED FORWARD BEND (5m), CAT-COW STRETCH VARIATION (5m)
Fri	SHOULDER ROLLS (5m), SHOULDER SHRUG STRETCH (5m), NECK ROTATION (5m)	SEATED HAMSTRING REACH (5m), DYNAMIC CALF ELEVATIONS (5m), BUTTERFLY INNER THIGH STRETCH (5m)	GENTLE CORE TWIST (5m), CHILD'S POSE SIDE STRETCH (5m)
Sat	TRICEP STRETCH (5m), WRIST FLEXOR STRETCH (5m), SHOULDER ROLLS (5m)	SIDE CLAMSHELL MOVEMENT (5m), GROUND-TOUCH FORWARD BEND (5m), GENTLE PIGEON POSE (5m)	SEATED TWIST STRETCH (5m), MODIFIED BOAT POSE (5m)
Sun	Rest	Rest	Rest

Week 3

Day	Upper Body	Lower Body	Core & Balance
Mon	SHOULDER ROLLS (5m), NECK TILTS (5m), TRICEP STRETCH (5m)	UPLIFTING BRIDGES (5m), GENTLE PIGEON POSE (5m), SEATED HAMSTRING REACH (5m)	SEATED TWIST STRETCH (5m), CAT-COW STRETCH (5m)
Tue	NECK ROTATION (5m), SHOULDER SHRUG STRETCH (5m), WRIST FLEXOR STRETCH (5m)	BALANCED QUAD PULL (5m), DYNAMIC CALF ELEVATIONS (5m), SIDE CLAMSHELL MOVEMENT (5m)	GENTLE CORE TWIST (5m), SEATED FORWARD BEND (5m)
Wed	WRIST EXTENSOR STRETCH (5m), SHOULDER ROLLS (5m), NECK TILTS (5m)	CHAIR-BASED HIP OPENER (5m), BUTTERFLY INNER THIGH STRETCH (5m), GENTLE PIGEON POSE (5m)	MODIFIED BOAT POSE (5m), CAT-COW STRETCH VARIATION (5m)
Thu	TRICEP STRETCH (5m), NECK ROTATION (5m), SHOULDER SHRUG STRETCH (5m)	GROUND-TOUCH FORWARD BEND (5m), UPLIFTING BRIDGES (5m), SEATED HAMSTRING REACH (5m)	GENTLE CORE TWIST (5m), CHILD'S POSE SIDE STRETCH (5m)
Fri	WRIST FLEXOR STRETCH (5m), WRIST EXTENSOR STRETCH (5m), SHOULDER ROLLS (5m)	SIDE CLAMSHELL MOVEMENT (5m), BALANCED QUAD PULL (5m), DYNAMIC CALF ELEVATIONS (5m)	SEATED TWIST STRETCH (5m), EXTENDED COBRA POSE (5m)
Sat	NECK TILTS (5m), TRICEP STRETCH (5m), NECK ROTATION (5m)	GENTLE PIGEON POSE (5m), CHAIR-BASED HIP OPENER (5m), BUTTERFLY INNER THIGH STRETCH (5m)	CAT-COW STRETCH (5m), MODIFIED BOAT POSE (5m)
Sun	Rest	Rest	Rest

Week 4

Day	Upper Body	Lower Body	Core & Balance
Mon	NECK ROTATION (5m), SHOULDER ROLLS (5m), WRIST FLEXOR STRETCH (5m)	UPLIFTING BRIDGES (5m), GENTLE PIGEON POSE (5m), BALANCED QUAD PULL (5m)	GENTLE CORE TWIST (5m), SEATED FORWARD BEND (5m)
Tue	TRICEP STRETCH (5m), NECK TILTS (5m), SHOULDER SHRUG STRETCH (5m)	CHAIR-BASED HIP OPENER (5m), SIDE CLAMSHELL MOVEMENT (5m), SEATED HAMSTRING REACH (5m)	CAT-COW STRETCH VARIATION (5m), CHILD'S POSE SIDE STRETCH (5m)
Wed	SHOULDER ROLLS (5m), WRIST EXTENSOR STRETCH (5m), NECK ROTATION (5m)	DYNAMIC CALF ELEVATIONS (5m), BUTTERFLY INNER THIGH STRETCH (5m), GROUND-TOUCH FORWARD BEND (5m)	SEATED TWIST STRETCH (5m), MODIFIED BOAT POSE (5m)
Thu	NECK TILTS (5m), TRICEP STRETCH (5m), SHOULDER SHRUG STRETCH (5m)	GENTLE PIGEON POSE (5m), BALANCED QUAD PULL (5m), CHAIR-BASED HIP OPENER (5m)	EXTENDED COBRA POSE (5m), GENTLE CORE TWIST (5m)
Fri	WRIST FLEXOR STRETCH (5m), WRIST EXTENSOR STRETCH (5m), SHOULDER ROLLS (5m)	SIDE CLAMSHELL MOVEMENT (5m), UPLIFTING BRIDGES (5m), SEATED HAMSTRING REACH (5m)	SEATED FORWARD BEND (5m), CAT-COW STRETCH (5m)
Sat	SHOULDER SHRUG STRETCH (5m), NECK ROTATION (5m), TRICEP STRETCH (5m)	GENTLE PIGEON POSE (5m), BUTTERFLY INNER THIGH STRETCH (5m), DYNAMIC CALF ELEVATIONS (5m)	CHILD'S POSE SIDE STRETCH (5m), SEATED TWIST STRETCH (5m)
Sun	Rest	Rest	Rest

5.3 Expert Plan

Week 1

Day	Upper Body	Lower Body	Core & Balance
Mon	NECK ROTATION (6m), SHOULDER ROLLS (6m), TRICEP STRETCH (6m)	GENTLE PIGEON POSE (6m), DYNAMIC CALF ELEVATIONS (6m), BALANCED QUAD PULL (6m)	CAT-COW STRETCH VARIATION (6m), EXTENDED COBRA POSE (6m)
Tue	WRIST FLEXOR STRETCH (6m), NECK TILTS (6m), WRIST EXTENSOR STRETCH (6m)	CHAIR-BASED HIP OPENER (6m), SIDE CLAMSHELL MOVEMENT (6m), BUTTERFLY INNER THIGH STRETCH (6m)	MODIFIED BOAT POSE (6m), GENTLE CORE TWIST (6m)
Wed	SHOULDER SHRUG STRETCH (6m), TRICEP STRETCH (6m), NECK ROTATION (6m)	UPLIFTING BRIDGES (6m), GROUND-TOUCH FORWARD BEND (6m), SEATED HAMSTRING REACH (6m)	SEATED FORWARD BEND (6m), CHILD'S POSE SIDE STRETCH (6m)
Thu	SHOULDER ROLLS (6m), WRIST EXTENSOR STRETCH (6m), WRIST FLEXOR STRETCH (6m)	BALANCED QUAD PULL (6m), DYNAMIC CALF ELEVATIONS (6m), GENTLE PIGEON POSE (6m)	SEATED TWIST STRETCH (6m), CAT-COW STRETCH (6m)
Fri	NECK TILTS (6m), SHOULDER SHRUG STRETCH (6m), TRICEP STRETCH (6m)	SIDE CLAMSHELL MOVEMENT (6m), CHAIR-BASED HIP OPENER (6m), BUTTERFLY INNER THIGH STRETCH (6m)	GENTLE CORE TWIST (6m), EXTENDED COBRA POSE (6m)
Sat	WRIST FLEXOR STRETCH (6m), NECK ROTATION (6m), SHOULDER ROLLS (6m)	UPLIFTING BRIDGES (6m), SEATED HAMSTRING REACH (6m), GROUND-TOUCH FORWARD BEND (6m)	CHILD'S POSE SIDE STRETCH (6m), MODIFIED BOAT POSE (6m)
Sun	Rest	Rest	Rest

Week 2

Day	Upper Body	Lower Body	Core & Balance
Mon	TRICEP STRETCH (6m), SHOULDER SHRUG STRETCH (6m), NECK TILTS (6m)	GENTLE PIGEON POSE (6m), DYNAMIC CALF ELEVATIONS (6m), BALANCED QUAD PULL (6m)	EXTENDED COBRA POSE (6m), SEATED FORWARD BEND (6m)
Tue	NECK ROTATION (6m), WRIST EXTENSOR STRETCH (6m), WRIST FLEXOR STRETCH (6m)	SIDE CLAMSHELL MOVEMENT (6m), UPLIFTING BRIDGES (6m), CHAIR-BASED HIP OPENER (6m)	MODIFIED BOAT POSE (6m), CAT-COW STRETCH VARIATION (6m)
Wed	SHOULDER ROLLS (6m), TRICEP STRETCH (6m), SHOULDER SHRUG STRETCH (6m)	BUTTERFLY INNER THIGH STRETCH (6m), SEATED HAMSTRING REACH (6m), GROUND-TOUCH FORWARD BEND (6m)	CHILD'S POSE SIDE STRETCH (6m), GENTLE CORE TWIST (6m)
Thu	NECK TILTS (6m), WRIST EXTENSOR STRETCH (6m), NECK ROTATION (6m)	BALANCED QUAD PULL (6m), SIDE CLAMSHELL MOVEMENT (6m), DYNAMIC CALF ELEVATIONS (6m)	SEATED TWIST STRETCH (6m), CAT-COW STRETCH (6m)
Fri	SHOULDER SHRUG STRETCH (6m), TRICEP STRETCH (6m), SHOULDER ROLLS (6m)	GENTLE PIGEON POSE (6m), CHAIR-BASED HIP OPENER (6m), UPLIFTING BRIDGES (6m)	EXTENDED COBRA POSE (6m), SEATED FORWARD BEND (6m)
Sat	WRIST FLEXOR STRETCH (6m), NECK TILTS (6m), NECK ROTATION (6m)	SEATED HAMSTRING REACH (6m), BUTTERFLY INNER THIGH STRETCH (6m), GROUND-TOUCH FORWARD BEND (6m)	MODIFIED BOAT POSE (6m), GENTLE CORE TWIST (6m)
Sun	Rest	Rest	Rest

Week 3

Day	Upper Body	Lower Body	Core & Balance
Mon	SHOULDER ROLLS (6m), NECK TILTS (6m), TRICEP STRETCH (6m)	UPLIFTING BRIDGES (6m), GENTLE PIGEON POSE (6m), SEATED HAMSTRING REACH (6m)	SEATED TWIST STRETCH (6m), CAT-COW STRETCH (6m)
Tue	NECK ROTATION (6m), SHOULDER SHRUG STRETCH (6m), WRIST FLEXOR STRETCH (6m)	BALANCED QUAD PULL (6m), DYNAMIC CALF ELEVATIONS (6m), SIDE CLAMSHELL MOVEMENT (6m)	GENTLE CORE TWIST (6m), SEATED FORWARD BEND (6m)
Wed	WRIST EXTENSOR STRETCH (6m), SHOULDER ROLLS (6m), NECK TILTS (6m)	CHAIR-BASED HIP OPENER (6m), BUTTERFLY INNER THIGH STRETCH (6m), GENTLE PIGEON POSE (6m)	MODIFIED BOAT POSE (6m), CAT-COW STRETCH VARIATION (6m)
Thu	TRICEP STRETCH (6m), NECK ROTATION (6m), SHOULDER SHRUG STRETCH (6m)	GROUND-TOUCH FORWARD BEND (6m), UPLIFTING BRIDGES (6m), SEATED HAMSTRING REACH (6m)	GENTLE CORE TWIST (6m), CHILD'S POSE SIDE STRETCH (6m)
Fri	WRIST FLEXOR STRETCH (6m), WRIST EXTENSOR STRETCH (6m), SHOULDER ROLLS (6m)	SIDE CLAMSHELL MOVEMENT (6m), BALANCED QUAD PULL (6m), DYNAMIC CALF ELEVATIONS (6m)	SEATED TWIST STRETCH (6m), EXTENDED COBRA POSE (6m)
Sat	NECK TILTS (6m), TRICEP STRETCH (6m), NECK ROTATION (6m)	GENTLE PIGEON POSE (6m), CHAIR-BASED HIP OPENER (6m), BUTTERFLY INNER THIGH STRETCH (6m)	CAT-COW STRETCH (6m), MODIFIED BOAT POSE (6m)
Sun	Rest	Rest	Rest

Week 4

Day	Upper Body	Lower Body	Core & Balance
Mon	NECK ROTATION (6m), SHOULDER ROLLS (6m), TRICEP STRETCH (6m)	GENTLE PIGEON POSE (6m), DYNAMIC CALF ELEVATIONS (6m), BALANCED QUAD PULL (6m)	CAT-COW STRETCH VARIATION (6m), EXTENDED COBRA POSE (6m)
Tue	WRIST FLEXOR STRETCH (6m), NECK TILTS (6m), WRIST EXTENSOR STRETCH (6m)	CHAIR-BASED HIP OPENER (6m), SIDE CLAMSHELL MOVEMENT (6m), BUTTERFLY INNER THIGH STRETCH (6m)	MODIFIED BOAT POSE (6m), GENTLE CORE TWIST (6m)
Wed	SHOULDER SHRUG STRETCH (6m), TRICEP STRETCH (6m), NECK ROTATION (6m)	UPLIFTING BRIDGES (6m), GROUND-TOUCH FORWARD BEND (6m), SEATED HAMSTRING REACH (6m)	SEATED FORWARD BEND (6m), CHILD'S POSE SIDE STRETCH (6m)
Thu	SHOULDER ROLLS (6m), WRIST EXTENSOR STRETCH (6m), NECK TILTS (6m)	BALANCED QUAD PULL (6m), SIDE CLAMSHELL MOVEMENT (6m), DYNAMIC CALF ELEVATIONS (6m)	SEATED TWIST STRETCH (6m), CAT-COW STRETCH (6m)
Fri	NECK TILTS (6m), SHOULDER SHRUG STRETCH (6m), TRICEP STRETCH (6m)	GENTLE PIGEON POSE (6m), CHAIR-BASED HIP OPENER (6m), UPLIFTING BRIDGES (6m)	EXTENDED COBRA POSE (6m), SEATED FORWARD BEND (6m)
Sat	WRIST FLEXOR STRETCH (6m), NECK ROTATION (6m), SHOULDER ROLLS (6m)	SEATED HAMSTRING REACH (6m), BUTTERFLY INNER THIGH STRETCH (6m), GROUND-TOUCH FORWARD BEND (6m)	MODIFIED BOAT POSE (6m), GENTLE CORE TWIST (6m)
Sun	Rest	Rest	Rest

Chapter 6: Focused Routines

As you delve into this chapter, it's essential to understand its unique offering in contrast to the weekly plans provided earlier. While the weekly plans are your comprehensive guide to holistic stretching, designed to be followed day-by-day, the routines in this chapter serve a specialized purpose.

The Distinction:

1. **Weekly Plans**: Think of these as your "core curriculum." They're structured, progressive, and meant to be followed in sequence. Each day's exercises aim for all-round improvement, ensuring different parts of the body are catered to throughout the week.

2. **Focused Routines**: These are your "electives" or "special modules." Each routine targets a specific need or time of the day. Whether you're looking to kickstart your morning with zeal, wind down for a serene night, or address a particular concern like pain or posture, these routines are your go-to.

While there might be some exercises common to both, their placement and purpose vary. In the weekly plans, they fit into a broader strategy, while in these routines, they're tailored to a specific outcome.

You can integrate these routines into your weekly plans. For instance, even if you're on Week 2 of the Intermediate Plan, you can still incorporate the "Morning Stretch Routine" upon waking up. It's all about listening to your body and recognizing what you need on any given day.

Now, let's embark on these focused routines, starting with a routine that's perfect for early risers - the Morning Stretch Routine

6.1 Morning Stretch Routine

Good morning! Are you feeling a bit stiff after a restful night's sleep? It's completely normal. As we age, our muscles and joints can sometimes feel a bit rigid after hours of inactivity. But, I've got a solution for you—a morning stretch routine designed specifically to kick-start your day.

Starting your day with these stretches isn't just about loosening up; it's about setting a positive, proactive tone for everything that follows. Consider this routine as your morning coffee for the muscles and mind—a way to perk up, increase your circulation, and get ready for the day ahead.

Now, you might be wondering why a morning routine is so crucial. Well, think of it as a gentle nudge for your body, signaling it's time to get moving. Plus, it's a lovely little moment of self-care, a way to check in with yourself before the day's hustle begins.

Here's your morning wake-up call, a series of exercises to get you moving and feeling great:

1. **NECK TILTS** - Wake up those neck muscles and ease any overnight stiffness.
2. **SHOULDER ROLLS** - A great way to loosen up the upper body and prepare for the day.
3. **CAT-COW STRETCH** - Activate your spine and engage your core.
4. **GENTLE PIGEON POSE** - A soft hip opener to address any tightness.
5. **DYNAMIC CALF ELEVATIONS** - Get those lower legs ready for the day's walks.
6. **SEATED FORWARD BEND** - A full-body stretch that emphasizes the back and legs.
7. **WRIST FLEXOR STRETCH** - Especially beneficial if you're planning to do any writing or typing.

Remember, take each stretch at your own pace and make sure you're comfortable. If something doesn't feel right, it's okay to skip it or modify. The key is consistency and tuning into how your body feels.

6.2 Pain Relief Routine

Pain is a word we all wish to erase from our lives, especially as we age. As our bodies undergo wear and tear over the years, it's not uncommon to feel discomfort in various areas. While there are numerous medical treatments and medications available, stretching is a natural, non-invasive way to alleviate some of that pain.

This Pain Relief Routine is meticulously designed to target common areas of discomfort in seniors, such as the lower back, neck, shoulders, and hips. But remember, it's not just about doing these stretches when you're in pain. Consistent practice can act as a preventive measure, potentially reducing the frequency and intensity of future discomfort.

Before we delve into the exercises, a word of caution: If any stretch intensifies your pain or feels wrong, stop immediately. It's essential to listen to your body and differentiate between a good stretch and harmful pain. Moreover, if you suffer from chronic pain or have a specific medical condition, it's a good idea to consult with a physician or physiotherapist before attempting these stretches.

Exercises for the Pain Relief Routine:

1. **NECK TILTS** - Often, pain originates from stiffness in the neck. Gentle tilts can release that tension.
2. **CAT-COW STRETCH** - This dual-move is a savior for the spine, especially the lower back.
3. **GENTLE PIGEON POSE** - Ideal for sciatica pain and tight hips.
4. **CHILD'S POSE STRETCH** - A resting pose that alleviates back and neck pain.
5. **SEATED FORWARD BEND** - Stretches the entire back and can relieve tension in the spine.
6. **SUPINE KNEE TWIST** - Helps in relieving lower back discomfort.
7. **CHAIR-BASED HIP OPENER** - Focuses on hip pain, offering gentle release.
8. **GROUND-TOUCH FORWARD BEND** - Stretches the back, hamstrings, and calves, all areas prone to pain.

Each exercise should be held for about 30 seconds to a minute, ensuring you breathe deeply throughout. The focus is on gentle, prolonged stretches rather than intensity. With time and regular practice, you might find this routine to be a natural painkiller, easing your discomfort and enhancing your quality of life. Remember to always prioritize comfort and safety over pushing your limits.

6.3 Flexibility Improvement Routine

Flexibility isn't just about being able to touch your toes or twist your body like a gymnast. As we age, maintaining and improving flexibility becomes crucial, not just for athleticism but for daily activities. Greater flexibility can mean the difference between reaching that high shelf with ease or depending on others. It can mean bending down to tie your shoes without a struggle or moving about without that nagging stiffness.

The Flexibility Improvement Routine focuses on elongating muscles, increasing the range of motion in joints, and ensuring that your body remains agile and supple. This is especially important for seniors, as improved flexibility can decrease the risk of injuries, reduce pain, and improve balance.

Before starting this routine, it's essential to understand that flexibility doesn't improve overnight. It requires consistent effort, patience, and, most importantly, regular practice. However, over time, you'll undoubtedly notice improvements, not just in flexibility but in your overall well-being and ease of movement.

Exercises for the Flexibility Improvement Routine:

1. **NECK ROTATION** - Enhances neck mobility and relieves stiffness.
2. **SHOULDER ROLLS** - Loosens the shoulder joints and increases the range of motion.
3. **SEATED TWIST STRETCH** - Great for spinal flexibility and abdominal stretching.
4. **BUTTERFLY INNER THIGH STRETCH** - Targets the inner thighs, promoting flexibility in the legs.
5. **GENTLE CORE TWIST** - Stretches the obliques and mid-section.
6. **SEATED HAMSTRING REACH** - Focuses on the hamstrings and lower back.
7. **BALANCED QUAD PULL** - Increases the flexibility of the quadriceps and hip flexors.
8. **WRIST FLEXOR AND EXTENSOR STRETCHES** - Ensures wrist joints remain mobile, essential for tasks like writing or opening jars.

As you practice this routine, always remember to breathe deeply and steadily. Aim for holding each stretch for about 30 seconds to a minute, allowing the muscles to gradually release and lengthen. Over time, as your flexibility improves, you might find daily activities becoming more effortless and enjoyable. The world seems a bit brighter when you can move freely within it!

6.4 Bedtime Stretch Routine

When the day's hustle and bustle winds down, and it's time to prepare for a peaceful night's rest, your body deserves some gentle attention. The moments right before sleep are an excellent opportunity to release tension, relax your muscles, and calm your mind. A bedtime stretch routine can serve as a bridge between the active parts of your day and the tranquil hours of rest.

This routine isn't about building strength or even improving flexibility; it's about finding tranquility. Stretching before bed can increase blood flow, reduce nighttime aches, and even improve the quality of your sleep. Moreover, it's a time to connect with your body, appreciate it, and prepare it for rejuvenation.

Exercises for the Bedtime Stretch Routine:

1. **CHILD'S POSE STRETCH** - A grounding stretch that allows for deep breathing and relaxation of the back muscles.

2. **SEATED FORWARD BEND** - Helps release tension in the back and hamstrings, while promoting calmness.

3. **GENTLE PIGEON POSE** - Opens up the hips and allows for relaxation in the lower body.

4. **NECK TILTS** - Releases any tension carried in the neck from the day's stresses.

5. **EXTENDED COBRA POSE** - Gently stretches the abdominal muscles and lower back, promoting relaxation.

6. **CAT-COW STRETCH VARIATION** - Serves to soothe and massage the spine after a day's activities.

7. **SUPINE KNEE TWIST** - Relaxes the spine and allows for a gentle rotation, releasing any tension.

Before beginning, set the mood. Dim the lights, play some soft background music if you like, and maybe even light a scented candle. As you move through each exercise, focus on your breathing – deep, slow, and rhythmic. Imagine each breath carrying away the day's stresses. When you've finished the routine, you should feel a deep sense of relaxation, paving the way for a restful night's sleep. Sweet dreams!

6.5 Posture Improvement Routine

In our modern world, many of us spend hours each day hunched over computers, looking down at smartphones, or sitting in vehicles and on couches. Over time, these habits can lead to a forward head posture, rounded shoulders, and a slouched upper back, commonly known as "poor posture." Not only does this affect our appearance, making us seem less confident and more fatigued, but it can also lead to back pain, reduced lung capacity, and other health issues.

Thankfully, with regular attention and the right exercises, it's possible to improve one's posture and reverse some of these adverse effects. This routine is designed to target the muscles responsible for maintaining an upright, confident, and healthy posture.

Exercises for the Posture Improvement Routine:

1. **SHOULDER ROLLS** - Loosens the shoulder joints and activates the upper back, teaching the shoulders to sit back and down.

2. **EXTENDED COBRA POSE** - Engages the muscles of the lower back and opens the chest, combating the effects of hunching.

3. **CHAIR-BASED HIP OPENER** - Opens the hips and counteracts the effects of prolonged sitting.

4. **CAT-COW STRETCH** - Mobilizes the spine, promoting a neutral posture.

5. **SEATED TWIST STRETCH** - Strengthens the obliques and other muscles responsible for an erect posture.

6. **SHOULDER SHRUG STRETCH** - Relieves tension in the trapezius, a common area of tightness for those with poor posture.

7. **TRICEP STRETCH** - Opens up the shoulder joint, allowing for a more upright posture.

Remember, while this routine can significantly aid in improving posture, it's also crucial to be mindful of your posture throughout the day. Every so often, take a moment to adjust your posture, pull your shoulders back, and ensure your spine is in a neutral position. Over time, with consistent effort and the support of this routine, you'll notice a difference not just in how you stand, but in how you feel. Stand tall and embrace the world with confidence!

6.6 Stress Relief Routine

Life today is rife with sources of stress: from work pressures to personal challenges, and the ever-present hum of technology. Our bodies often carry this stress in the form of muscle tension, particularly around the neck, shoulders, and back. Over time, this tension can lead to physical discomfort and exacerbate feelings of anxiety and unease.

Stretching, with its emphasis on deep breathing and focused movement, can be a wonderful antidote to stress. This routine is crafted to relieve tension, promote relaxation, and provide a momentary escape from the daily grind. Engaging in these exercises can act as a reset button, helping you approach challenges with a clearer mind and a calmer spirit.

Exercises for the Stress Relief Routine:

1. **NECK TILTS** - Aids in releasing tension in the neck, where many of us hold stress.
2. **CHILD'S POSE STRETCH** - A grounding exercise that stretches the back and offers a moment of introspection.
3. **SEATED TWIST STRETCH** - Helps to wring out tension in the mid-back and spine.
4. **GENTLE CORE TWIST** - A subtle movement that massages the abdominal organs and promotes relaxation.
5. **CAT-COW STRETCH** - A fluid motion that engages the spine and reminds us to move with ease and grace.
6. **RHYTHMIC TOE TAPS** - Brings attention to the feet, grounding us and diverting our focus from stressors.
7. **EXTENDED COBRA POSE** - Opens the chest, promoting deeper breathing and a sense of openness.

As you go through each exercise, focus on your breath. Deep, rhythmic breathing can enhance the stress-relieving benefits of stretching. Let each inhale bring clarity, and each exhale release tension. By the end of this routine, you'll hopefully feel a weight lifted, ready to face the world with renewed serenity and strength.

6.7 Energy Boosting Routine

There are moments in everyone's day when energy dips and motivation wanes. It could be that mid-morning slump, the post-lunch lethargy, or the evening fatigue. While it's tempting to reach for a cup of coffee or a sugary snack, there's a healthier, more holistic way to reinvigorate yourself: stretching.

This routine is designed to get your blood flowing, awaken your senses, and give you that much-needed burst of energy. These stretches are dynamic, helping to stimulate the cardiovascular system, increase oxygen flow to the brain, and activate major muscle groups. It's like giving your body and mind a natural jolt, sans caffeine.

Exercises for the Energy Boosting Routine:

1. **DYNAMIC CALF ELEVATIONS** - These not only engage the calves but also promote circulation throughout the legs.

2. **GENTLE PIGEON POSE** - A great way to open the hips and get the blood flowing more freely.

3. **SEATED HAMSTRING REACH** - Stretches the back of the legs and encourages good posture.

4. **HEEL-FOCUSED WALKING** - Activates the foot muscles, providing a grounding sensation.

5. **MODIFIED BOAT POSE** - Engages the core, promoting stability and a burst of energy.

6. **SHOULDER ROLLS** - Loosens tension in the shoulders and neck, areas which can inhibit energy flow when tight.

7. **NECK ROTATION** - Encourages circulation to the head, helping to clear any mental fog.

Whenever you find yourself dragging, take a few minutes to run through this routine. It's a quick way to recharge, making you feel more alert and vibrant. Remember, sometimes the best way to invigorate the mind is by moving the body. Give it a try and experience the natural energy surge for yourself.

Chapter 7: Tips and Techniques

Embarking on a stretching journey, especially in our golden years, is not just about going through the motions. It's about embracing an approach that marries the mind, body, and soul. This chapter is dedicated to providing you, our cherished reader, with invaluable advice to optimize your stretching routines. Whether you're a novice or a seasoned stretcher, understanding the nuances of stretching can greatly influence the results you reap. From the rhythm of your breath to tuning into your body's whispers, let's dive into the subtleties that can elevate your stretching experience.

7.1 Breath Control during Stretching

Breathing is an innate act, something we do without conscious thought from the moment we're born. However, when integrated with intentional movements, such as stretching, the role of breath transforms from being merely functional to profoundly therapeutic. In the realm of stretching, especially for seniors, understanding and practicing controlled breathing can greatly amplify the benefits of each stretch.

The Power of Breath in Stretching

Breathing deeply and consistently during stretches helps deliver oxygen-rich blood to your muscles. This not only aids in muscle relaxation but also promotes healing and reduces muscle fatigue. Furthermore, focusing on your breath can act as a form of meditation, helping you remain present during your routine and enhancing your overall sense of well-being.

Techniques for Breath Control

1. **Diaphragmatic Breathing (Belly Breathing):** This technique involves deep breathing through the diaphragm rather than shallow breathing from the chest.
   - *How to Practice:* Lie down comfortably. Place one hand on your chest and the other on your abdomen. Breathe in slowly through your nose, letting your abdomen rise (your chest should remain still). Exhale slowly through your mouth, pressing down gently on your abdomen. This helps in engaging core muscles and deepens the stretch.
2. **Rhythmic Breathing:** Synchronizing your breath with your movements can enhance the effectiveness of each stretch.
   - *How to Practice:* If you're moving into a stretch, inhale as you begin the movement and exhale as you deepen into the stretch. The exhale can aid in relaxation and allow you to stretch a bit further.

3. **Paced Breathing:** This involves taking slow, controlled breaths. Pacing can help manage any discomfort during a stretch and keep you calm.

   - *How to Practice:* Inhale for a count of four, hold for a count of four, and then exhale for a count of four. Adjust the count as per your comfort.

Benefits of Breath Control

- **Enhanced Muscle Relaxation:** As you focus on your breathing, your muscles tend to relax, which can lead to a deeper and more effective stretch.
- **Reduced Risk of Injury:** Controlled breathing ensures you're not holding your breath, which can lead to increased blood pressure and tension.
- **Mental Clarity and Focus:** Focusing on your breath can help clear your mind, reducing distractions and enhancing your stretching session's overall quality.

Embracing these breathing techniques might seem a bit overwhelming at first, especially if they're new to you. However, with consistent practice, they'll become second nature. Remember, it's a journey, and each breath you take is a step toward a more flexible, relaxed, and invigorated you.

7.2 Holding Times and Repetition

As you delve deeper into your stretching journey, understanding the nuances of how long to hold a stretch and how often to repeat it becomes pivotal. Holding times and repetitions aren't just arbitrary numbers; they're tailored recommendations that help ensure you're reaping the full benefits of each stretch without risking injury. Especially for our senior readers, these elements offer a roadmap to better flexibility and muscle health.

The Importance of Holding Times

The duration you hold a stretch matters significantly. It's during this holding period that your muscles, tendons, and ligaments get the chance to relax, lengthen, and adapt.

- **Short Holds (10-15 seconds):** Ideal for a quick refresh, these stretches can be incorporated throughout the day to combat stiffness, especially if you've been stationary for a while.
- **Medium Holds (20-30 seconds):** This is the most common duration recommended for most stretches. It's long enough to allow the muscles to fully relax and lengthen without causing strain.
- **Long Holds (60 seconds or more):** Reserved for deep stretches, this duration is typically for advanced practitioners or when supervised by professionals. It allows for profound muscle relaxation and flexibility enhancement.

Repetition Matters

Repeating a stretch multiple times can enhance its effectiveness. Here's why:

1. **Increased Muscle Memory:** Repeating a movement aids in muscle memory, helping the body become more accustomed to the stretch over time.

2. **Progressive Muscle Relaxation:** With each repetition, you might find you can stretch a little deeper, as the muscles become more relaxed and pliable.

3. **Enhanced Blood Flow:** Repeating stretches ensures a continuous flow of blood to the region, promoting healing and reducing muscle fatigue.

Recommendations for Seniors

- **Frequency:** For most stretches, repeating them 2-3 times provides an optimal balance between effectiveness and safety.

- **Rest Between Repetitions:** Give your muscles a brief break (10-15 seconds) between repetitions. This little pause allows the muscles to recover and prepare for the next round.

It's essential to remember that these are general guidelines. Everyone's body is unique, and what works for one person might not work for another. Always pay attention to how your body responds. If a stretch feels too intense or causes pain, it's crucial to ease out of it and, if needed, adjust the holding time or repetition. Your journey with stretching is personal, and it's about progress, not perfection. Always prioritize comfort and safety over pushing boundaries.

7.3 Listening to Your Body

In the world of stretching and exercise, there's a phrase that you'll often hear: "Listen to your body." While it may seem clichéd, its importance cannot be overstated, especially for seniors. Your body has its way of communicating with you, and it's crucial to heed its messages. By tuning into your body's signals, you can ensure that you're not only getting the most out of your stretches but also avoiding potential harm.

Understanding Your Body's Signals

1. **Comfort vs. Discomfort:** A proper stretch will often produce a feeling of slight discomfort—like a gentle pull. This is normal and indicates that the muscles are being extended. However, this discomfort shouldn't translate to pain. If you feel a sharp, stabbing, or intense pain, it's a sign to stop and adjust.

2. **Recognizing Fatigue:** It's natural to feel a bit tired after a good stretch, but excessive fatigue might indicate overexertion. Remember, it's okay to take things slow and break when needed.

3. **Heat and Sweating:** A little warmth in the muscles is good—it means blood is flowing. But excessive heat or sudden sweating might be signs to slow down or take a break.

Adapting to Feedback

- **Adjustment:** If a particular stretch feels too intense, try a milder version or reduce the holding time.

- **Alternatives:** Not every stretch is suitable for everyone. If one doesn't feel right, consider alternative stretches that target the same muscle group.

- **Consistency:** Regularly practicing stretching can help your body get used to the movements, making it easier to discern between good discomfort and potential pain.

The Power of Intuition

Over time, as you consistently engage in stretching exercises, you'll develop a heightened sense of intuition about your body's needs and limits. Trust this intuition. Sometimes, even if a book or instructor suggests a particular stretch, your body might resist it. And that's okay. Your personal experience is the best guide.

Final Thoughts for You

Dear reader, embracing the practice of stretching is not just about following steps or achieving a particular pose. It's a journey of understanding and respecting your body's unique rhythm and needs. As you age, this connection with your body becomes even more vital. Embrace the stretches, but more importantly, embrace the wisdom that your body offers. Remember, it's always communicating; all you need to do is listen.

Conclusion

As we draw this journey to a close, it's essential to reflect on the profound connection between stretching and the quality of life, especially for seniors. From the foundational principles of stretching to the nuanced techniques that amplify its benefits, every chapter in this guide was meticulously crafted to empower you on your wellness journey.

We began by understanding the very essence of stretching, especially its significance for seniors. Recognizing the pivotal role it plays in enhancing mobility, ensuring comfort, and promoting overall health, we delved into its myriad benefits. Safety, of course, took precedence, ensuring that each movement respects the unique needs and boundaries of the senior body.

Our exploration of the human anatomy was thorough, compartmentalizing stretches to target the upper body, lower body, and the core. This systematic approach ensures a holistic stretching routine, leaving no muscle group unattended. Each exercise was chosen not only for its efficacy but also for its feasibility, especially for seniors.

The 4-Week Stretching Plan was an embodiment of progression. Starting as a beginner, moving to an intermediate level, and finally embracing expert routines, the plan is a testament to the idea that growth is continuous. It emphasizes that age is not a limitation but an avenue for new learning.

Our focused routines, be it the invigorating morning stretches or the calming bedtime ones, are tailored to address specific needs and moments in a day. They serve as reminders that stretching isn't just a physical activity; it's a way to connect with oneself, be present in the moment, and address the varied needs of the mind and body.

Lastly, the tips and techniques reiterated the importance of being attuned to one's body. Listening, understanding, and adapting—these are the cornerstones of a successful stretching routine.

To you, dear reader, remember that this book is more than just a guide; it's a companion. As you stretch, grow, and evolve, let the pages of this book be a constant source of inspiration and knowledge. Embrace the stretches, but also the journey of self-discovery they lead you on. With every twist, turn, and tilt, you're not just working on your body; you're celebrating it.

Thank you for allowing this guide to be a part of your wellness journey. Stay stretched, stay vibrant, and always, always keep moving forward.

Index Exercises

Printed in Great Britain
by Amazon

42090593R00051